The Menopause

Deirdre Lundy was born in New York. After sitting the leaving certificate in Ireland, she went to University College Dublin, from where she was awarded a medical degree in 1987. She has practised in primary care in Ireland ever since, specializing in sexual and reproductive health, and particularly in women's health. She has worked extensively in the area of menopause care, as well as for many years teaching fellow doctors about the menopause with the Irish College of General Practitioners. She is also accredited by the British Menopause Society as a BMS menopause specialist and trainer. In 2021 she became clinical lead in Ireland's first dedicated menopause clinic at the National Maternity Hospital, Holles Street.

Deirdre lives in south Dublin with her family.

The Menopause

The Essential Guide to Managing Your Health in Mid-Life

DR DEIRDRE LUNDY

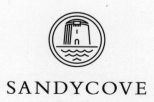

SANDYCOVE

an imprint of

PENGUIN BOOKS

SANDYCOVE

UK | USA | Canada | Ireland | Australia
India | New Zealand | South Africa

Sandycove is part of the Penguin Random House group of companies
whose addresses can be found at global.penguinrandomhouse.com.

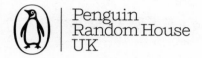

First published 2023
001

Copyright © Deirdre Lundy, 2023

The moral right of the author has been asserted

Set in 12/14.75pt Bembo Book MT Pro
Typeset by Jouve (UK), Milton Keynes
Printed and bound in Great Britain by Clays Ltd, Elcograf S.p.A.

The authorized representative in the EEA is Penguin Random House Ireland,
Morrison Chambers, 32 Nassau Street, Dublin D02 YH68

A CIP catalogue record for this book is available from the British Library

ISBN: 978–1–844–88614–2

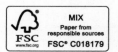

To the brave people who contacted RTÉ Radio 1's *Liveline* to speak out about menopause – for you and for every menopausal woman who left a doctor's office feeling worse than when she went in.

This is your book.

Contents

PART II
MANAGING THE SYMPTOMS OF
PERIMENOPAUSE AND MENOPAUSE

PART IV
MENOPAUSE AND PARTICULAR
HEALTH ISSUES

Introduction

The menopause and me –
an unlikely romance

Around 2004 I had started to skip periods but didn't pay much heed to it. Just another blip in the workings of the female body, which, let's face it, rarely runs like clockwork. I was a young woman, periods were a nuisance anyway, so what of it? I had no idea what was coming down the track. By April 2005 I was post-menstrual – done. I was just turning forty-four years of age.

I was out-the-door busy at that time. When I look back at my calendar now, I wonder how I did it: I had three kids with incredibly busy school and social lives, a husband who was trying to keep a family business alive during yet another economic nightmare, and I was working about six part-time jobs. I was working in a few different family planning clinics around Dublin. Then I started doing sessions down in the Bray Women's Health Centre as illness cover for a doctor there. Meantime, I was already teaching for the Irish College of General Practice and delivered most of their women's health educational events. I also taught medical students in the Royal College of Surgeons and in Beaumont Hospital. On top of all that I was running a household (a housekeeper has never seen the inside of my home!). Somehow, in the midst of all this, I muddled along and kept going. I was having lots of sweats and hot flushes, and my sleeping pattern was way off, so I put myself on a weak oral hormone replacement (HRT) drug, Livial, mainly because it was cheap – money was tight and it would not bring my periods back.

And so it went on – until it all came crashing in on me.

My actual memory of the beginning of the bad times is a bit hazy – but maybe that is a good thing? I have all my wall calendars for the last twenty-five years, though, and they helped me piece the sequence together. I have *Sick at work* written on my wall calendar for a day in the spring of 2009. That day was probably the turning point: I had been feeling a bit off over the previous few days; somewhat dizzy, a little light-headed. I was in the surgery and when I went to take blood from my patient (I can still remember her name, Aisling), my hands started to shake and I couldn't catch my breath. *What the heck is going on?* I thought. Nothing like this had ever happened to me before. I felt really scared and I had to stop what I was doing, which was humiliating and, of course, only added to my distress.

I explained to Aisling that I was feeling awfully ropey all of a sudden and it would not be safe for me to do the blood test. I suggested we should skip that for now and I would get her back in as soon as possible to complete the examination. She agreed. Why wouldn't she? God help her, she must have been terrified of being needle-stabbed by a shaky, swaying doctor! I'm still grateful for how kind she was that day.

Aisling left and I lay on the examination couch, hoping that whatever it was would pass quickly. I urgently tried to diagnose myself: I had had some focal migraines over the years – that is a migraine headache that starts off with neurological warning symptoms – and I had experienced some severe ones while pregnant, so I wondered could this be the start of another migraine? But I knew this was not typical. I usually got a funny visual thing (an aura, we call it) before the migraine struck, whereby the bottom right half of my field of vision would go off-kilter, like I was looking through broken glass. I had learned to recognize this warning sign and when it showed up, I would throw some paracetamol/Zomig/whatever-was-handy into me and close my eyes, and it would usually pass without too much drama. But this was not like anything I had experienced before, so I was worried.

I knew that people who get focal migraine are more at risk of getting a mini-stroke, so now I'm thinking, *Could I be having a mini-stroke?*

My mind was flying through all the possibilities. I was in no fit state to work, so a colleague kindly cancelled all my remaining patients that day and drove me home because I was simply unable to do so myself. I hit the bed, waiting for the migraine to kick in, telling myself over and over that I would be okay in a few hours.

I was shaky and nauseous and could not sleep. I don't know how the kids got home from school that day – I must have called my husband to get them, but I don't remember. I was glued to the bed. After a few hours I was no better. This was no focal migraine.

I felt okay enough by the next morning to go hiking as usual with my wonderful Ramblin' Roses buddies in my hill-walking group, but at one stage I had to be helped when I became dizzy and breathless. This was nuts. I rang my GP and booked the first appointment they could give me.

I remember that sitting in the waiting room was torture. When I was outside in the fresh air it wasn't so bad, but sitting in the cramped waiting room with people around me made me feel trapped and worried. I was obsessing over the notion that I would faint or do something else to embarrass myself. Looking back, I would now describe myself as having acute anxiety, but at the time – in the thick of it – I was scared and confused. Physician, heal thyself? No chance. I had no idea what was going on with me.

I saw a young doctor who took some blood and suggested rest until we got the results.

A week later I went back to the practice to see my usual GP. The blood test results were normal. We chatted and he gently explained that he thought this could be an anxiety-related thing. I immediately and loudly disagreed, telling him that 'I don't get anxiety!' (Boy, if I had a penny for every time a patient has said that to me.) He suggested that I speak to a bio-feedback practitioner – someone who assesses all the physiological processes going on in your body and can help you control them – who would assess my background levels of stress/anxiety. He told me that sceptics like me often found it useful. So, off I went.

The practitioner I went to see was lovely. She wired me up to the heart rate and BP and breathing monitor and we went through some questions about my day-to-day life. I scored 13/15 for background stress/anxiety. That was way too high, leaving no room for additional stressors, and something clearly needed to be done. She introduced me to cognitive behavioural-type therapy (CBT) and I went back to my GP for a prescription for anti-anxiety medication. I started to feel a bit better almost immediately, although that was probably because I had a name for this thing, people were helping me, and I was optimistic again.

I cannot convey how deeply disappointed I was in myself. I had allowed my mind to make me physically unwell to the point where I couldn't work. The shame. *I am strong, I don't let things get me down, I am the one who copes* – that was my precious self-image, and now it was all torn asunder. I felt like I had failed, and my sense of self was completely undermined as a result.

I should have taken some time off at that point, but I refused to be defeated by this 'nonsense' and was determined not to miss work. Yet I found that even driving to the surgery in Bray triggered anxiety, and I had to do guided breathing just to get into the clinic. A small piece of a low-dose Xanax helped enormously, but I was terrified of getting dependent on them – and I also worried that my GP would think less of me if I needed to go back and ask him for more. Instead, I rationed them out like tiny slivers of gold dust.

You can see that this situation was going nowhere fast. I was due to fly to France with the kids and my husband and his extended family, and I was secretly dreading it. I had developed a fear of flying, after years and years of not having a bother with it – a clue, you say. Anyway, a plane ride during this rotten episode was the last thing I needed, but the break was a good idea and I was always less anxious in familiar company than I was on my own or with strangers, so off we went. Although it was a good holiday and I did enjoy parts of it, I remember having to hold hands with my eight-year-old niece as we strolled around the shops – not for her comfort, but for mine.

The day after we returned home, I had to fly alone to London, and that was a nightmare. The perfectly normal flight was terrifying and I disembarked from it an anxious mess. I recall choosing to sit on the floor in the back of the meeting hall because I felt more 'grounded' there. What must people have thought?

After I got home from London, I made an appointment with a psychotherapist who, while pleasant, was not much use to me. I bought the self-help books he suggested and I did the exercises and I quickly began to realize the reality of the situation: *Yep, I am getting panic attacks, I have anxiety, I am vulnerable, I am not as clever as I thought I was. I am not superwoman. Shit!*

I did not cut back on work, of course – oh no, that wouldn't do for me, plus we badly needed the income. So, I just tried to avoid as many triggers as I could while trying to keep juggling all those balls. My husband used to take time off work to drive me to all the various evening and weekend lectures I gave. I avoided driving alone on the motorway at all costs – still do, to be honest – as it was a place I would regularly start to experience a panic attack. I was a bag of nerves and jitters, triggers and reactions, anxieties and maddening thoughts.

And so it continued, on and on, for eighteen long and lonely months, until eventually and quite serendipitously I found help. I was chatting to a good friend about my situation, and she recommended a different psychotherapist, and that woman changed my life. Let's call her Maud. Well, Maud was an angel, or she was my angel at least. We talked every week for months. She was so gentle and understanding, and I tried to embrace everything she said because I liked her and trusted her. I was so broken down after months and years of this crap that I was wide open to anything she had to say.

That day in the surgery with Aisling marked the beginning of my menopause symptoms. I was forty-seven years old. My periods had stopped four years previously and although I'd had some flushes and sweats, I thought I was fine. I had embarked on a bumpy journey and never even noticed when I was leaving port. I was a doctor and a woman, but I was clueless about my own body and brain. I was thick with symptoms yet didn't join the dots and recognize the big picture.

Not only that, but all along I was on a low-dose HRT treatment. However, as I often say to patients now, HRT is not a magic bullet. I assumed that as I was on HRT, there wasn't much more hormones could do for me. Obviously, I was way too young and too symptomatic for something as low dose as I was using. I used the anti-depressant/anti-anxiety medication my GP offered and was happy for it as I needed to claw back some quality of life for myself, but I look back and think how handy it would have been to have had a little nuanced HRT knowledge then, like I have now.

I am still prone to anxiety and must actively remember to be kind to myself. I tend to take on all the work that is offered and then get overwhelmed, still, to this day. Lots of people do this. I have learned to link my self-worth to how many paid events I have on the calendar. But I am trying to learn to say 'no' more often and not feel guilty. It is a journey, though. It took me sixty years to get this way, so it'll probably take the next sixty to unlearn some of those thoughts/feel-ings/body-symptoms/behaviours – but I am getting there.

Now, I see so many patients who remind me of me. I have learned to sense anxiety in other people at twenty paces. 'I can smell it off you,' I sometimes say, and they look shocked, but then usually relieved (mostly). I briefly tell them about my anxiety, and hope that helps open the door to a conversation.

So, while menopause was tough for me and I wasn't a great help to myself at the time, I can finally say that I am grateful for this life lesson. I'm also grateful for good doctors and therapists, great pharma-ceuticals, amazingly supportive family and friends, and the strength to drop the pretence. The truth is, none of us is as well as we want the world to think we are. We are all carrying more than anyone will ever know, and we all need a little help. That goes for menopause, for anxiety, for mental health, for physical conditions – for life, really. The absolute hardest part is accepting that you are not impervious to struggles, both physical and mental, getting over the embarrassment of it, and asking for help. I hope this book is of use to you in that regard.

My own menopause was a lot worse than it needed to be, I believe. In retrospect I shake my head and feel sorry for myself, but then I also know that I learned more from my own life than any 'mental health in primary care' lecture could ever convey. I think – I hope – that I have become a better doctor as a result of my own ill health and the struggle to find the right fix. And the upside of all that suffering was that it sparked a devoted interest in the whole subject. I fell for it in a big way, hence the unlikely romance. I'm in my early sixties now, but I'm still slap-bang in the menopause world, thanks to my work.

For a long time I have wanted to write a comprehensive menopause handbook for women. The science is actually pretty simple and the knowledge is there. The silence that has long enveloped 'the change' has led to misinformation, embarrassment and a complete inability to just talk like grown-ups about vaginas and wombs and periods and all the stuff that can get dismissed as 'women's things'. That drives me nuts. It's just bodies, it's all natural, and the help is sorely needed, so why not be upfront and to the point and just *talk*?

So that's what we're here to do, talk openly and honestly about the menopause – including perimenopause and post-menopause – and give reliable information rooted in scientific evidence and the medical literature, and using up-to-date data and guidelines from the European Menopause and Andropause Society (EMAS), the British Menopause Society (BMS), the British Medical Association (BMA), the Australasian Menopause Society (AMS), the UK's National Institute for Health and Care Excellence (NICE) and the International Menopause Society (IMS). You'll find website addresses for all of these in the resources section at the back of the book. There are hundreds of medical publications on the menopause, some are useful and important, others are rubbish. I do not have the training to read and interpret the information from every last publication, so I rely on reliable guidance from the menopause societies. These are groups of experts who are committed to reading all the literature, reviewing all the studies, and providing doctors and their patients with comprehensive and up-to-date information. Their work is the solid basis for mine.

The important thing to realize is that the menopause is a whole-body phenomenon that affects every major organ, including the brain. It's physical and it's psychological. The menopause is like a big chrysalis that you step into, your whole self enters that chrysalis. What emerges can be wonderful, but you need to understand what's going on and work to your own benefit on this, to help yourself. And to do that, you need to have a solid understanding of what menopause is all about, which is what I want to give you here. Your experience of it will differ from everyone else's, it's a subjective thing, but when you have the tools to understand it and talk about it, you're in a great position to face up to it and handle it as well as you can. I want you to be your own best advocate. I hope this book helps you to do that.

What follows is a simple, logical progression from a complete explanation of what menopause is – that's the science part, with a full-on anatomy lesson, because you need to know what's going on 'down there' and 'in there'. I'm going to give you a guided tour of your vagina, so you know exactly what's going on with it. You don't get a mirror free with this book, but you will be coming face-to-face with your lady parts anyway.

After all that explanation, we'll look at how you'll know if you're in perimenopause, menopause or post-menopause. The dreaded symptoms!

We will examine the crucial question of how perimenopause and menopause are diagnosed, because I know this has been a source of great frustration for so many women. When it comes to discussing it with your GP, to identifying symptoms and interpreting them properly for your body, you need to be on the ball with that. We'll look at that process in detail. You'll have all the correct terminology, which will give you a head start when you go to talk about your experiences with your GP or nurse or whoever. You don't want to be muttering about being in 'the time of life', bogged down in euphemisms. I want you to be confident that you know what you're talking about – and that you understand what they're talking about, and can ask questions.

And then there are the different routes into menopause. Some of you will have a 'natural' menopause, triggered by aging, but for many people menopause can arrive early, caused by medical treatment (iatrogenic) or premature ovarian insufficiency (POI), for example. We'll look at those scenarios separately.

I'll set out the management options – both non-medical and medical. There's plenty you can do to help smooth the path for yourself without pharmaceuticals, and we'll look at all of those. Although I, for one, am going to be buried with my HRT patch firmly in place – I am never giving that stuff up, if I have a choice.* So, I can give you first-hand experience on that as well as the medical science.

---

* My role models in this regard are a couple of eighty-plus-year-old patients who always came to see me together, coming down on the train from Donegal. They were great friends and they made a yearly pilgrimage to Dublin for a day of shopping, lunch and a trip to the menopause doctor! They had been on HRT since their forties and they wanted to stay on it. No doctor in their area would prescribe it for them any more, even though they had weaned themselves down to the tiniest of doses anyway. I always looked forward to seeing them, these two happy and healthy seniors, living their best life, and my attitude was: *Who am I to pull that carpet out from under them?* Besides, their prescription was fully in keeping with the NICE guidelines, which state that it is not up to the doctor to say when or if to stop HRT – the individual decides. Those ladies must be passed on by now, I guess (otherwise they would both be well over a hundred years old!), but I miss them and aspire to be like them.

Though we doctors talk all the time about 'treating' menopausal symptoms, it would be more accurate to talk about 'managing' your menopause. This is because every menopause experience is individual, each lasts for its own period of time, which is entirely unpredictable, and each requires its own optimal way to manage the set of symptoms that the experience brings. It's a case of figuring out what your symptoms are and how severe they are, what your medical and family history means for your choices on how to handle it, your own preferences in terms of medication (if you decide to go down that route), and what you want it to achieve for you, and the length of time you stay on it.

Transitioning from having an abundance of ovarian hormone to having nearly none takes years, can be much harder on some people than others, and is far from predictable. You can have good days and bad days, good months and bad months, it varies hugely from person to person. So, management of your menopause process needs to be tailored to fit you.

All of this is based on my own experience, but also – and more importantly – on more than thirty-five years of clinical experience. I've been talking with women about their menopause for a long time, listening to their personal experiences, prescribing for their particular needs, charting the course of their transition right along with them. I've learned so much. Although I gotta tell you, when it comes to being a menopause doctor, it's half medical science and half witchcraft – it's so unpredictable and subjective an experience, that those of us involved in diagnosis and treatment sometimes have to use creative problem-solving and intuition – yours and ours! – alongside the robust medical data, to hit on just the right solution for any given patient.

It was my dream as a little girl growing up in New York to one day be a doctor. I came to Ireland as a seventeen-year-old, sat the Leaving Cert, trained in UCD and have been practising medicine here for over thirty-five years. I have been lucky enough to have wandered into an area of health care that I really enjoy.

As you can imagine, it's fascinating and very fulfilling. And I'm very heartened by the progress I've seen in Ireland over the past ten years. At the start, women would sidle in the door, literally whispering their story to me, as if a bolt of lightning might strike them dead for even saying the words 'menopause' or 'vagina' out loud. But that has slowly changed, and I'm delighted to see that women have found the confidence to speak out. More and more patients are happy to share the intimate details of what's going on with them, and they seem far more comfortable asking for help to improve their genital and sexual health. For example, lots of ladies have mentioned to me that they find anal sex more comfortable than vaginal sex after menopause. *Fair play*, I say to them – *but let me help fix your vagina too, please, and give you an even broader repertoire*. I think it's really beautiful that women are discussing the issues openly with their sexual partners and finding their own solutions. That's a definite and positive change in attitude. And it's the kind of menopause response I like to hear about – forthright, honest, grown-up, needs-based and a tailor-made personal solution.

I am always gathering and regurgitating information on reproductive health; mainly because I love it, but it helps me keep up to date for my patients and it is an essential part of my other work as a medical educator. In fairness, I do like talking, and over the last ten years I have become more and more involved in delivering medical talks and seminars on women's health around Ireland. There has been quite a growing interest among GPs and GP nurses, particularly in menopause management, and pre-Covid I spent many weekends travelling around Ireland delivering talks on how to better serve menopausal patients. My good friend and superlative GP colleague Dr Nicola Cochrane dubbed me the 'Radiant Goddess of the Menopause' at one stage, and I gladly accepted the title!

The options for managing menopause-related symptoms really took a terrible nosedive in 2002, after an infamous study and the highly flawed interpretation of its findings misled people into thinking that HRT caused breast cancer (see Chapter 9). It didn't then and it doesn't now, and it was so sad to witness the needless suffering among so many ladies who were terrified of trying anything related to HRT to alleviate their symptoms.

The pendulum started swinging back towards common sense with the 2015 publication of a document on menopause management by NICE that finally put to rest the exaggerated fears and negativity surrounding the use of menopause hormones. Now, instead of news-papers and television scaring the crap out of everyone, the popular press was announcing how great it was not to have to suffer bad meno-pause symptoms any more, declaring that 'HRT is good for you again' – like, it never wasn't. As I specialized in menopause care in the private clinic I worked at in Bray, I got lots of hands-on experience as the demand for HRT started to climb after 2015.

An extraordinary series of programmes on RTÉ Radio 1's *Liveline* in May 2021 – when caller after caller shared heartbreaking stories of struggling with debilitating symptoms – brought the topic of menopause out of the closet in Ireland forever. This was followed by considerable positive momentum regarding menopause education in health care in Ireland. The HSE's National Women and Infants Health Programme had already been looking at improving meno-pause care, among many other unmet areas of women's health, and in November 2021 we got plans under way to roll out the first of many hospital-based, public Menopause Speciality Clinics in Ireland. I was honoured to be asked to be the lead for the first clinic to open, based in the National Maternity Hospital, Holles Street, ably assisted by Dr Nicola Cochrane and our dynamo of a Clinical Nurse Manager, Claire McElroy.

I have written guidelines and handbooks for doctors and nurses on the menopause and HRT, but I was never tempted to reach out to non-medics before. It's harder to write for the general public than for doctors, nurses, pharmacists, physios, et cetera, because we all know the fancy terminology and the secret handshakes and all the other weirdness that makes 'medical-speak' so unintelligible and impene-trable. I have tried my best to make the information in here both accurate and accessible without talking down. I hope you find some-thing in here for you.

Deirdre x

PART I

So, you think you're menopausal?

1. What is the menopause?
And why the hell is it happening to me?

Well, now, these are good questions. There is often a lot of confusion as to what constitutes 'menopause', so this is a good starting point for us, to give some specific definitions for perimenopause, menopause and post-menopause. This chapter will define these terms in relation to natural menopause, which means a change in hormones that occurs naturally as we age. This isn't the case for everyone going through menopause, of course. There are many people dealing with induced menopause for one reason or another. We will discuss their menopause experience in Chapters 6 and 7. But here, for our first look at what the menopause actually is, we'll chart a course through the natural lifecycle of our hormones, from before birth to post-menopause.

Part of the confusion among some health-care professionals, and no doubt among the patients who are trying to figure it all out, is that the word 'menopause' often means different things to different people, which can cause lost-in-translation moments when we are discussing it. So, bear with me here as we sort it out, and apologies if this feels like a biology lesson. (You can take heart from knowing that doctors themselves hate the female cycle pictogram and all those labels and stages – because it's so complicated!)

Starting with the basics – the womb, the ovaries and the ova (eggs)

The womb is a small bag of stretchy muscles that is shaped like an upside-down avocado. The middle of it is hollow and the lining of the hollow bit is made up of special tissues that are designed to entertain a pregnancy, should that need ever arise. The ovaries are the main players when it comes to menopause. They are a pair of juicy-looking, almond-sized glands that are tucked into the pelvis, usually on either side of the womb. The ovaries store all the eggs needed for reproduction (about 500,000 eggs by the time a girl starts menstruating) and they are also the source of many essential hormones, including the three key female reproductive hormones, or *sex hormones* as we call them: the *oestrogens*, the *androgens* and natural ovarian *progestagen* (known as *progesterone*).

Puberty, which usually hits between the ages of ten and twelve, is the time of your life when the eggs in the ovaries, the womb and all the other reproductive structures start to get ready for fertility and periods and the hope of a pregnancy. This is a huge moment because that is what life on earth is focused on – reproduction of the species. It's what we are made to do, to keep the human species going.

Hormones, puberty, menstruation, pregnancy and menopause all happen in the womb and the ovaries, but they are organized by hormones made in the control centre of the female brain: the hypothalamus and the pituitary gland. This is the key point for everything we are going to discuss about the menopause – *it is all about the hormones*. Hormones are the source of everything that is happening in your body, when we talk about menopause. If the hormones aren't playing ball, things go awry very quickly.

In puberty, the hypothalamus and the pituitary gland of the brain start to release their own signalling hormones in a unique way. This causes the ovaries to kick in for real and they start to release their sex hormones in a very structured, complex, monthly cycle. This is the start of puberty and it's what causes the eggs to ripen, to hopefully mature and be released, and to eventually end up either as a pregnancy or as part of a menstrual bleed (period). Naturally, this is a big change in a child's life and can bring on lots of disruption. Even when this symphony of hormones and ballet of eggs/periods/ pregnancy is working well, it can be challenging. Puberty is a rocky time for most kids. The conductor of the whole performance are the hormones, which is why the correct term for puberty is the *hormonal maturation process*.

The hormones that run your life

The main hormones that are required to give a female human her reproductive ability are: follicle stimulating hormone (FSH), luteinizing hormone (LH), estradiol (E2) and progesterone (P). These are the hormones that are responsible for the monthly menstrual cycle and healthy, successful pregnancies, if we are lucky enough to have them.

The reproductive hormones work in concert with the sex hormones to control your menstrual cycle (see pages 152–3 for a day-by-day rundown). Like I said, a symphony. In fact, these four principal hormones – follicle stimulating hormone, luteinizing hormone, estradiol and progesterone – really run your life, up to a point. Not only do they control your monthly cycles, but they also play a significant role in how you feel and how you think, and some people struggle with some of the effects of those hormones. For example, oestrogen is generally a feel-good hormone, but not all women get some mood elevation from it. It's also notorious for causing negative symptoms, such as swelling in the breasts, which is why cyclical breast pain is quite common for some people. Oestrogen can also have an impact on blood vessels, so higher levels of oestrogen and headache can be related. Similarly, while it is an essential reproductive hormone, progesterone can cause swelling in the tissues and can have a mood-lowering impact for some people if the levels are going up and down, as they do in a menstrual cycle.

Sometimes it is the balance between amounts of oestrogen and progesterone in the blood and in the tissues that can cause good and bad effects in the body. *Balance* is the key word here. Achieving balance between oestrogen and progesterone is a big part of coming to terms with having female biology. Most of us muddle through happily enough, we get used to our 28-to-35-day cycles with their rises and falls of oestrogen and progesterone. But it's very much an individual and subjective experience. And it can change from month to month as well, just to keep us on our toes.

During our reproductive life we will usually release only about 400 eggs in total, during 400 periods. By the time we are about forty years old, we usually have anywhere from 1 to 10,000 eggs left, and although it's now less likely, we are still capable of having a pregnancy. If we follow the numbers, it implies that we could go on having periods until seventy years or older, but it doesn't happen like that, and we don't really know why for sure. But a few decades after puberty we hit the perimenopause. This is when the symphony starts to hit some bum notes and the ballet dancers decide they don't want to dance any more – probably because their knees are giving out. It can be a cacophonous mess!

So, although we don't actually run out of eggs as such, they do seem to have a limited shelf life, and usually by fifty to fifty-five years of age the eggs are no longer viable and the ovaries decline and shrivel a bit – no more juicy almonds – and they become more like tiny, shrivelled, defunct raisins. I know some of the menopausal ladies are rolling their eyes and thinking, *Yep, shrivelled, that sounds about right!*

The end of the menstrual cycle

I mentioned above that we don't know why the female reproductive cycle plays out like this, but there are some theories as to why we stop having periods and cease to be able to reproduce in our fifth decade. It's a distinct difference between males and females. When a young man hits puberty, he experiences the maturation of the developing testicles, which then start to produce sperm and the main male sex hormone, testosterone. Men produce sperm and testosterone for the rest of their lives. There is a definite decline, but it never stops completely. So why aren't their female counterparts made like this?

It is thought that some mammals are evolutionarily enabled to have older, post-reproductive females in the tribe/community who can help with hunting/gathering/child-rearing without being compromised by pregnancy/childbirth/breastfeeding, all of which are a drain on personal resources and not without risks. This makes some sense, as there are many other 'long-lived' species that, like us, seem to have a time limit on childbearing. I like this quote from Dr Jared Diamond, a physiologist at the University of California: 'menopause, like big brains and upright posture, is among the biological traits essential for making us human.' A case of 'it takes a village', I imagine. But others would argue that senior females are not the only members of a community who can assist with child-rearing duties, therefore the hypothesis is somewhat limited.

An alternative theory is that becoming post-menopausal is a relatively new phenomenon. Personally, I am inclined to buy this one. It is likely the case that our ovaries have always worked for about fifty years and then shut up shop, but what is new is that we are living much longer lives now. Since 1900, most populations are living longer because of better public health measures, socio-economic conditions, along with a little help from modern medicine. For example, in the 1850s in Massachusetts, which holds the earliest census data for the USA, life expectancy at birth for 'free-living white women' was forty years of age. No post-menopause for most of those privileged ladies!

What is new in modern times is that menopause is not a precursor to the end of our lives, as it once was, but instead is the beginning of a new chapter – and hopefully a great chapter where we can enjoy the fruits of career and family and whatever life we've set up for ourselves. Yes, some of us will be more fortunate than others at this time, and it's far from plain sailing, but I have to say that I like this perspective on menopause and think it's helpful. Anyone who lives long enough to experience menopause can consider themselves very lucky. It wasn't always so, and you'll have friends and acquaintances who don't make it that far. You lived through puberty and survived – now you get to go through another major life transition and find out what's on the other side.

The menopause is actually a single day!

So, back to the search for solid working definitions of the menopause process. One of the names we give to it is 'the change', which is a way to cover it up in polite conversation but is also accurate in its own way because menopause is when the familiar rhythm of our menstrual cycle and the hormones that control it start to change. Women begin to lose their ovarian function and ultimately it all just stops. The journey from having lots of eggs and lots of pregnancy-promoting hormones to having none at all is commonly referred to as 'the menopause'. So, you'll hear people say that they are 'going through the menopause' and we all nod and know what they're talking about. But if you say that phrase to a bunch of gynaecologists, they will need to ask some questions to find out what you mean. This is because, in gynaecology circles, the term 'menopause' is defined as the last day of your last menstrual period. Menopause comes from the Greek words *meno* (monthly) and *pausis* (pause or stop), so it means the day menstruation stopped for good. If a gynaecologist says, 'She is menopausal,' they mean her periods have ceased. Gynaecologists can only identify when this has happened when they can look back at the last twelve months and say, 'Oh wow, you have stopped having periods.' Not very high tech!

When we assess someone and discover their last ever period was over twelve months ago – and they are not pregnant or on some medication to artificially stop their bleeds – we define them as 'post-menopausal'. This is an important medical distinction. It lets us know who is and is not at risk of getting pregnant, which is important when we are prescribing medicines and discussing contraception. It lets us know who should and should not be experiencing vaginal bleeding, which is also extremely important. If a person is designated as post-menopausal, we expect to see different things when we do ultrasound scans, hormone blood tests, et cetera.

You can see where the ongoing confusion arises with the term 'menopause'. Most non-medical people use the word to describe the transitional time in a person's life when they go from having regular cycles and fully functional ovaries to when it starts to decline and eventually stops. The correct term for this process is 'the climacteric', but only a handful of people use that term. You hear people say, 'I am in the menopause,' or, 'I have menopause symptoms.' I'd lay a bet that you've never heard anyone say, 'I am in the climacteric.' You might think they'd bought a new car if you heard that!

Many months or years before your last period, your ovaries will start to release female hormones in a different way. Some days the ovaries will release the normal amount of sex hormone, some days they will release too little or too much. It is this *hormonal fluctuation* that starts off the symptoms of the menopause and is known as the climacteric. Blood tests of sex hormone levels can often be normal when people are in the climacteric, so the diagnosis is usually made by symptoms alone.

To get around this loose use of terms, and the fact that 'the climacteric' is relatively unknown and not used outside of health care, a new phrase was added to the menopause lexicon, which is the now-familiar 'perimenopause'. Again, the average person might use this interchangeably with menopause, or they might use it to mean 'I'm on the edge of full-blown menopause' – it's never really been strictly defined. But for our purpose we need proper definitions, so let's nail down the perimenopause now.

The perimenopause means you are in transition, experiencing hormone fluctuation symptoms but still getting regular or occasional periods, which may be quite irregular or heavy or painful. This is a new word, but it's a legitimate word and is recognized by most menopause health care practitioners, so we'll use it throughout this book. It's a handy way to separate out the process towards stopping (perimenopause), the moment of stopping (menopause), and the time after periods have stopped completely (post-menopause).

Charting the end of the menstrual cycle

The three 'stages' are useful in discussing the process of menstruation and the menopause, but they don't line up neatly with the symptoms of the transition from full ovary function to no ovary function, which is what everyone and his sister now calls menopause. There are no hard and fast rules here, no timeline that I can hand you and you can plot out your life by it. Wouldn't it be great if we could pin it to specific ages and be nicely prepared and then tick it off when each stage is done? But no, that's not how it happens. All I can tell you is what it involves, how it's diagnosed, the symptoms and the various ways available to you to deal with it, from HRT to exercise. But within that, you'll need to listen to your own body and chart your own periods and give yourself as much information as possible, so that you know what you're dealing with as each symptom and phase occurs.

The key thing, from a gynaecological point of view and from your health point of view, is the status of the menstrual cycle. This tells you where you are on the spectrum. So, if you are still menstruating – even from time to time, or quite predictably, or regularly but then with gaps – all of that is considered perimenopausal, meaning that your body is winding down its reproductive capability, but you are still more than able to get pregnant by accident, so you must use precautions if you're not keen for a pregnancy. If you are still having any kind of menstrual cycle, you have not hit menopause. And this state of winding down but not yet having stopped, which we are calling perimenopause, can last anywhere from five to ten years. Again, there's no schedule on it, it just is what it is for your own body.

The most common time for a woman in the developed world to finish her menstrual cycle permanently is around fifty-one or fifty-two years of age (although many women finish earlier than that). However, it's not impossible to meet people who bleed quite regularly well into their middle to late fifties, although it's rare, so you shouldn't be worried if you're an older woman and still get periods – that's perfectly acceptable.

When the stuttering menstrual cycle finally putters out, that's it – menopause. You'll realize this afterwards, by checking the calendar and seeing your last red X marking the day you had your final period. It's always a good idea to keep a period diary, but particularly so in your forties and fifties. The day will come when you'll have your very final period, and then you're out and through.

A woman who no longer gets menstrual periods, no longer gets monthly bleeding, is identified as post-menopausal. As I said, this is an extremely important medical designation because it means there should be no more vaginal bleeding and if there is, that is a big, big red flag to your GP or gynaecologist. We would get very concerned about that and would need to rule out cancer, first and foremost. When you need to be vigilant is if you haven't had a period for at least a year and you're over fifty years of age, and then you start bleeding again, particularly if that bleeding is heavy or unpredictable. This can be an early warning sign for cancer of the womb-lining, so it's essential to get it checked out. Now, loads of non-cancerous things can cause bleeding symptoms as well, such as polyps, fibroids, STIs – they can all produce weird bleeding – but we only go looking for those other causes after we have ruled out cancer of the womb-lining. So, when I write a letter to the gynaecology clinic asking for a patient to be reviewed, the top priority, the first appointments, are always saved for the women whose periods were meant to be gone forever but who have started to bleed again.

Can a woman like that, a woman whose periods are well over, still have menopause-related symptoms? Yes, she can. Can a woman whose periods were well over and then came back again (so she needs to have investigations for womb-lining cancer) still be getting menopause-related symptoms? Yes, she can, but she is called a post-menopausal woman by the gynaecology clinic. The symptoms and the stages don't necessarily match up – and it's important that you know that.

KEY TAKEAWAYS

- Menopause is the last day of the last menstrual period you will ever have.

- Perimenopause is the years leading up to menopause, as the amount of female hormone being released by the ovaries starts to change and as a result you experience changes in what was normal for your body and/or how you feel.

- Post-menopause is your life after menopause when you no longer have a cycle of menstrual bleeding.

- The key when it comes to hormones is balance. Menopause robs you of hormonal balance for a while, and you might need help to artificially balance the hormones until your body has fully adjusted and made the transition to being post-menopausal. Some women may need help in balancing their hormones for the rest of their lives.

- Whatever is going on with your periods, you can have menopause symptoms quite badly and may need some help – and that help might well be HRT. Sadly, many GPs, gynaecologists and other doctors believe, and tell patients, that you cannot be in the menopause if you are still having periods – NOT TRUE!

2. How will you know?

Figuring out where you are on the menopause spectrum

You might be expecting this to be the longest chapter in the book, given the sheer number of symptoms that can be attributed to menopause. The root of the problem is that sheer number – I've seen lists with fifty symptoms on them – and also the uniqueness of each person's experience, the individuality of onset and ending – just the range of unpredictables and possibles that come with it. That means it's difficult to give you a neat package of symptoms that link to a diagnosis.

The symptoms, whichever ones you experience, will stem from the brain and the ovaries, where the hormones reside. They are caused by hormonal imbalance initially and then, later – after the age of about fifty-five to sixty – by hormonal decline. (Although this does not apply to people whose ovary hormones are impacted by gynae surgery, chemo, radiation, et cetera.) As your ovaries wind down, they not only start to pop out eggs less efficiently, but they also become less organized when it comes to hormone production. That's the cause of all your misery right there.

Some people will experience this transition very acutely, with severe, life-altering symptoms, and others will have a very mild experience. It is hard to predict how your own menopause will go until you get there and start feeling it. Some evidence suggests that your mother's or sisters' experiences might give you a hint as to how your menopause will go, but many other factors will also play a role. A big one is smoking. If you are a smoker, some sources suggest it can make your menopause symptoms – particularly the hot flushes and sweats – much worse.

The symptoms are so varied, and there are no blood tests that confirm the diagnosis – I'll explain this in the next chapter – so it can be tricky to be sure that all the symptoms a patient is describing are in fact menopause and that there isn't something else going on. Some symptoms are obvious – like flushes and sweating. Some are more subtle – especially the changes in mood, a lack of confidence, and the feeling of being unable to cope. That is why speaking to a menopause-knowledgeable doctor can be so helpful at this time of your life.

So, what are the symptoms to look out for? I'll give you the most common symptoms I encounter when meeting patients. Some of these can be linked to other health problems, so we cannot simply assume that everything that starts happening to a woman in her forties and fifties is menopause. But when we see one or two of these symptoms in an otherwise healthy person who has no family history of disease that might be linked to similar symptoms, and who has normal blood tests, scans, et cetera, then it is almost always menopause-related. And if the symptoms ease off when we do a trial of HRT, it is even more likely to confirm a diagnosis of perimenopause. Thankfully, most of us do not get all of the following symptoms – that would be a nightmare! – but even one or two of these, if severe and persistent, can cause an awful loss of quality of life, and need to be sorted out.

These are some of the little messengers that bring you the good news that you are in the perimenopause:

- hot flushes and night sweats
- sleep disturbance and tiredness
- emotional and cognitive issues like low mood or mood swings, irritability/anger, anxiety, poor memory, poor concentration, a cloudiness in thinking (many women call it 'brain fog')
- palpitations, dizziness, headaches
- heavier periods, or skipped or irregular periods
- loss of elasticity in the vaginal walls and loss of lubrication: this can make things like exercise, getting a smear test and having vaginal sex less comfortable for some women
- a decline in sex drive: low libido and/or difficulty achieving orgasm
- a decrease in metabolism: leading to increase in weight and obesity
- a loss of muscle mass (known as sarcopaenia)

- as some women move deeper into the transition, issues to do with declining collagen levels can become noticeable (collagen is a protein in the body that is used to make connective tissue), so weakness of the pelvic floor can begin or disimprove
- bladder issues: urgency (needing to rush to the loo), frequency (peeing too often), painful urination, frequent urinary tract infections (UTIs), leakage of urine and wetting yourself
- skin, hair and nail quality decline as collagen levels drop even further, leading to thinning hair, loss of head hair, skin issues, itchiness and crawling sensations (known as formication)
- joint complaints: aches and pains, poor exercise tolerance
- restless legs, which can seriously impair sleep.

The amount of distress a symptom can cause and the impact that symptom might have on your life will, of course, vary from person to person. Emotional symptoms, in particular, can cause confusion for the patient and the GP as some people are dealing with anxiety, low mood, irritability/rage, and yet are still having periods. These women are often offered mood drugs as a first-line attempt at helping them regain some balance when, in fact, hormone therapy would usually be the more effective way to manage those symptoms.

Blood tests are often taken during a menopause consultation, but if you have been having periods recently, it is likely you will have reproductive hormone levels in the 'normal' range – but that does not mean you are not perimenopausal. Many women with typical, profound menopause symptoms have 'normal' ovarian hormone levels. When I do blood tests for women with perimenopause/menopause symptoms who are still bleeding, I will usually be looking for other causes of symptoms, like thyroid hormone, haemoglobin levels, et cetera, and not reproductive hormones. As we will see in the next chapter, the diagnosis of menopause for people over the age of forty to forty-five is usually made by the symptoms alone and does not need any confirmatory blood tests (in line with NICE and BMS guidance).

The BMS does recommend we look at female hormone levels for women under forty-five, and particularly under forty, who are exhibiting symptoms of perimenopause, as these would be women with a potential diagnosis of early or premature menopause, respectively.

Now the treatment will be the same, but I think the narrative is slightly different: if you get perimenopause symptoms after the age of forty to forty-five and you would *like* HRT, then go for it; if you are in an early or especially a premature perimenopause, you *need* HRT because you are at far greater risk, and so we will push hard to encourage you to replace that lost oestrogen with HRT, because you are too young to be without it.

Menopause and its symptoms are clearly no picnic, and some ladies suffer much worse than others. The good news is that the worst of the symptoms usually tail off by your late fifties to mid-sixties; the bad news is that some women continue to have troubles well into their sixties and beyond. I'm sorry to have to tell you that. But, on the other hand, there is much you can do to mitigate and manage your symptoms, so medicine is here to help.

Hot and bothered – the best-known symptom of menopause

I suppose the one symptom that the world at large is most aware of when it comes to perimenopausal symptoms would be the hot flushes and sweats, or as we call them, the vasomotor symptoms.* Why do these occur? We're back to oestrogen, of course. Normally in a female with regular, fertile, healthy hormone levels, small changes in the core temperature of the body, where the organs are located, will not cause a noticeable change in the temperature of the surface of our body. This is because sensors in our skin blood vessels learn to ignore small changes in core temperature. Oestrogen plays a large role in this blood vessel stability. But when oestrogen levels start to become unpredictable or change outside of their normal rhythm, the stability of the blood vessels in the skin on the surface of the body becomes vulnerable to core temperature changes in such a way that even small increases of the core temperature can cause quite drastic increases in the surface temperature of our body – and this can happen many, many times in a day.

* The term 'vasomotor' relates to the action of the body's blood vessels or its *vascular* system.

For me, my flushes were very profound. I would feel a sort of tingling and a suffusion of sensation, usually starting around my knee-caps, and then it would rise up towards my pelvis, my belly, my chest, into my neck and up to my face and the top of my head. Sometimes it was so severe that it would take my breath away. At first, it was quite frightening because I wasn't sure what exactly was happening to me. Then I got way too used to it, until I was a veteran of that horrible sensation. A few seconds after that suffusion, that tingling, that tidal wave sensation rising up through me, the sweating would start. This was my body trying to release the excessive surface heat – just like it would if I had gone for a run or if something had frightened me. My surface temperature would shoot up and I'd start to sweat, sometimes profusely.

I usually noticed the sweating predominantly on my lower back, the top of my lip, and especially under my eyes. If I was wearing make-up or close-fitting clothes, there would be a visible stain and the make-up would be visibly running. Sometimes my face would be red and people would say to me, 'Are you okay? You don't look well, would you like a drink of water?' So, alongside the anxiety I was feeling, there was the embarrassment in public as well. With the embarrassment, the anxiety and the physical disruption all running full-tilt, I'd end up worrying that I was actually experiencing the beginnings of a heart attack. I'd be thinking, *Maybe this is what angina feels like? I don't know. Maybe I'm having a stroke? My grandmother had mini-strokes. I'm a little young, but who the hell knows?* Of course, that cycle of worry and anxiety drove the sweating and the heat further, causing even more discomfort. And this could happen to me once an hour, twice an hour, completely unpredictable. It was absolutely horrible during the day, out in public, although eventually I did kind of get used to the fact that the sensation would come and go and I wouldn't die. That was a bit reassuring.

I also hated it at night-time. It would happen in the middle of the night, when I was sound asleep, lying in my bed and wearing as little as possible to keep cool, the window open, a fan on, and yet in spite of all that, several times a night I'd go through the same process. I'd wake up to the physical sensation of the sheets beneath me being soaking wet, the pillowcase too, and I'd have no choice but to get out of the bed, lay down a towel, change what I was wearing, push the window open even further . . . but nothing could prevent it from happening.

And then you're also disturbing the sleep of the person lying next to you. No fun.

Now picture this happening when you also perhaps have family members, be it elderly relatives or young children, who also can disturb your night's sleep, and that's going on night after night after night. The impact that night sweats and flushes can have on a person's well-being is incalculable. It's not dangerous in itself, but it is so disruptive and a real killer when it comes to your quality of life. This is no doubt why night-time symptoms are among the most notorious aspects of the perimenopause. Thankfully, though, they are one of the many things that we have the most tools to improve and change, but you need to be able to access a doctor who knows how to manage these symptoms.

Feeling blue – mood changes

The number two symptom on the 'hotlist' (sorry!) of very well-known symptoms is mood changes. Generally, when I'm giving a lecture to doctors and nurses on the menopause, I talk about the physical symptoms separate from the emotional symptoms, but I think it's important to recognize both equally. Most doctors and nurses will recognize the physical symptom of a flush or a sweat for what it is – it's the perimenopause – but a lot of times a woman in her forties or fifties will come in to discuss the onset or worsening of mood issues, and I have found that very often health-care providers fail to recognize mood changes as one of the most common presentations of the perimenopause. As I said before, oestrogen in general is a stabilizing and mood-elevating hormone, which is why, when oestrogen levels are at their highest, i.e. during pregnancy, some women are said to 'glow'.

Most, but not all, women find that their mood is quite good during pregnancy, but then soon after giving birth, when oestrogen levels plummet back towards the typical level, that decline in oestrogen can bring on quite a profound mood drop. Many women will experience the four-day 'Baby Blues', when they become tearful and anxious after having a baby or a late miscarriage. Worse still is post-natal depression, which can be a significant psychological disorder. This is the same process: you were flying high on a wave of oestrogen and then that wave dropped and you are left feeling low and depleted. Well, that is what happens in perimenopause, too. All of this is triggered by the hormone changes, mainly the oestrogen decline, that are distinct characteristics of perimenopause.

Is it any wonder that mood and mood changes can be a big part of your menopause experience and impact your quality of life? I think this is something many people don't realize – that hormonal imbalance is a really big deal that brings physical, psychological and emotional symptoms. When our hormones are out of whack, it affects our entire system. I know people joke about women and moodiness, but it's actually very serious because a person can lose their enjoyment of life when their mood hits the skids. This is why the whole understanding of and response to the stages of menopause must be focused on working to achieve better hormone balance. That's the key to managing the symptoms.

The other hormone that plays a big role, as we already know, is progesterone. The levels of progesterone in our bodies are responsible for maintaining the lining of the womb and getting it ready for pregnancy – hence *pro-gest*, as in gestation. When those levels start to build after the egg is released, early in the menstrual cycle, until they crescendo the day before you bleed, your premenstrual mood can be very disrupted because progesterone is largely a mood-lowering hormone. It is the hormone thought to be responsible for premenstrual syndrome (PMS) – once known as premenstrual tension (PMT) – and premenstrual dysphoric disorder (PMDD) – an extreme form of PMS.

Some women find it very hard to tolerate the rising levels of progesterone in the second half of their cycle, and only really breathe and get their life back when the bleed finally arrives, which signals the drop in progesterone. Then they can look forward to a couple of days, a week, maybe two weeks of relatively good mental and physical health until the progesterone levels start to rise again. As you can imagine, women who are vulnerable to PMS will also be vulnerable to the relative fluctuation in oestrogen and progesterone that happens during the perimenopause.

We also can't forget that there is a whole other group of people who suffer from mood disorder, whether it's inherited through their family or because of traumatic disruptive experiences in their life, among other things. Not everybody enjoys good mood, and if you have mood disorder, you'll know about it – usually from your teens or early twenties. You may have struggled for a long time with this, and then the perimenopause hits. This can be a very challenging time because while you may have developed coping mechanisms or found therapies and medicines that have helped to manage your mood vulnerability in younger life, the internal disruption of the perimenopause can really throw you for a loop. You might find that what used to work to improve your mood may no longer help.

So, what I am really trying to say here is that mood changes in the perimenopause can come seemingly out of nowhere and surprise you – they can hit you right out of left field. (I use that baseball metaphor all the time, but I don't really know why something coming out of left field is such a surprise to baseball players!)

You might be experiencing low mood or mood changes or anxiety, with or without panic episodes, for the first time in your life and be feeling bewildered, like a stranger to yourself. You might have struggled with mood your entire adult life and now it worsens, threatening your sense of self and your ability to cope, and you feel that you are not managing it as well as you once did. This is a chicken-and-egg thing: you can have primary mood disruption from the hormone fluctuation of the perimenopause and/or you can have secondary mood disruption, which is a further disruption and perhaps worsening of a pre-existing mood issue due to the hormonal changes taking place in your body.

It is very important to be aware of this aspect of perimenopause and menopause so that you can recognize it for what it is and stay calm in yourself when handling it. Remember, too, that it's a perfectly normal reaction to the hormonal changes that are occurring. When hormones rise or drop, we are deeply affected. You can't change that fact. We can treat it, yes, but you need to know that hormonal imbalance is very real and affects everybody. You aren't different, or weak, or silly, or overreacting. You are in a body that is transitioning from being reproductive to non-reproductive, and that can generate pretty huge symptoms. Of course it can, it's a massive physiological change. So, go easy on yourself, forgive yourself for being human, and try to get the help you need to manage those hormones as best you can.

The timeline of menopause

Of course, every woman is different, but there has been some useful research conducted into the timeline of perimenopause and menopause – most notably the 2001 Stages of Reproductive Aging Workshop (STRAW), carried out in the USA.

The STRAW criteria provide an excellent overview of how we experience reproductive aging as we approach menopause. While I object to pigeon-holing women as such (I am in the STRAW Stage 4d of my menopause, by the way!), it does help to give you a sense of the journey that is the peri/menopause. The researchers divided a woman's life into three main stages:

- **reproductive** (subdivided into early, peak, late and later)
- **menopausal transition** (subdivided into early and late – and known by us as perimenopause)
- **post-menopausal** (subdivided into earlier, early, late and later).

The stages of the womb's lifecycle are tracked according to the status of the menstrual cycle. So, in the Reproductive stage, the menstrual cycle is 'variable to regular' in Early, it is 'regular' in Peak and Late, and then changes to 'Subtle changes in flow/length' in the Later stage. In the Reproductive stage, there are no menopause symptoms.

In the Menopausal Transition (Perimenopause), things start to kick off. In the Early stage, the menstrual cycle is classed as 'variable length', with persistent seven-day difference in length of consecutive cycles. No one bleeds exactly every twenty-eight days – there is usually a few days of variation in what we would call a 'regular' cycle. But when your period starts coming more than seven days late or more than seven days early, that means you have a symptom of early perimenopause.

In the Late stage, there is amenorrhoea, which means no menstruation. This remains the case for the Post-menopause stage, naturally. They note that vasomotor symptoms like hot flushes are characteristic of Late Perimenopause and Early Post-menopause, so they can hang around for quite a while.

And then in Late Post-menopause you get more symptoms of uro-genital atrophy, in other words the bladder and urethra areas (uro) and the vulva, vagina, cervix and womb areas (genital) can start to slouch off and not work so well. If this gets really bad, it can lead to atrophy, which basically means decay. Not a nice thought.

You can see, then, that they're not going by your age here, instead they look at your menstrual cycle and your symptoms and classify your stage of menopause that way, which makes sense.

Your menstrual cycle is taken as the key measure, but that is backed up by your hormone levels. The main hormones – FSH, AMH, Inhi-bin B – are all Low in the first two stages, then drop to Very Low in Post-menopause. And the number of egg-containing follicles in your ovaries does the same: the follicle count is Low in Reproductive and in Perimenopause, and then drops to Very Low in Post-menopause. Those counts will confirm that you are moving towards menopause, once your menstrual cycle has made the first announcement.

The STRAW researchers say that this expected timeline of the menopause transition applies only to 'typical' women. They added special subsections on women with other medical conditions or characteristics that would affect their timelines, such as the following.

- *Cigarette smoking and being overweight/obese*: while smoking and high BMI (body mass index) may influence hormonal levels and the timing of the perimenopause, the report notes that these should not change the menopause journey characteristics.
- *Polycystic ovary syndrome (PCOS) and premature ovarian insufficiency (POI)*: the report freely admits that people with PCOS or POI (which are discussed in Chapter 6) may not necessarily fit into their model. POI refers to premature or early menopause, and the diagnosis of POI may be trickier to make, especially for: women who have had surgical procedures to treat or investigate heavy or abnormal periods, including hysterectomy, dilation and curettage (D&C), endometrial ablation (melting away the inner layer of the womb-lining with lasers or radio-waves or local heat); and for women on

combined hormonal contraceptives. The report gives a special mention to women with severe chronic illnesses or women undergoing chemotherapy, noting that a significant proportion of women who need cancer treatment, particularly with alkylating agents (a common type of old-school chemotherapy that damages the DNA of rapidly growing cells), may experience episodes of perimenopause symptoms and might even have a rise in their FSH and a drop in their AMH levels and follicle counts, only to have it all slip back to normal again.

- *HIV*: women living with HIV may not fit neatly into this scheme; many of these women seem to experience symptoms of the perimenopause at a younger age, and their symptoms can be more severe. But if their viral load is low or they have good immunological control, then women with HIV should proceed through their menopause transition just like anyone else.
- *Tamoxifen and aromatase inhibitors (AI)*: women who are using these medications do not fit the STRAW staging because FSH and estradiol levels may be impacted by Tamoxifen and AI, plus you can get abnormal bleeding when on Tamoxifen. This means the STRAW menstrual bleeding prediction is no use to us in these cases.
- *Surgical removal of one ovary and/or a hysterectomy*: the study has NO data on the impact of removal of a single ovary and/or hysterectomy on the expected perimenopause-to-menopause timeline. We may have to wait for STRAW +20 for that data. That update was due in 2021, by the way, but – thank you, Covid – there's no sign of it yet (in mid-2022).

How long can this keep going on?

Right now, you're probably thinking, *How the hell long does this thing last?* It's all individual, so there's no strict timeline for these symptoms. They can kick off up to a decade before you stop bleeding. It is hard to predict how long you might be troubled by menopause symptoms – things like your own genes, your past health problems and certain lifestyle factors will all play a role. It is not uncommon to have two to five years of noticeable symptoms that will eventually just improve and disappear, but it is also not uncommon for patients to say they are still experiencing sweats and flushes well into their late fifties and sixties.

There are two triggering issues at work here – the fluctuation of the hormones, and then the lack of the hormones. Once you stop bleeding – which you can generally expect to happen around the age of fifty-one or fifty-two, or soon after – your hormone levels will measurably start to fall. This can make your symptoms much worse for a time but then, eventually, after as many as five years or so, most of those symptoms will dwindle as your body finds its new natural rhythm, particularly those symptoms likely caused by a change in hormone levels.

I have heard it said that a woman in her mid-sixties has less female hormone in her blood than a teenage boy. This makes a lot of sense as some of the symptoms of the menopause seem to be more related to the changing levels of hormone than to hormone loss. Flushes, for example, are more related to fluctuating levels than they are to hormone loss altogether, so it's very common for women to get flushing and sweating in the early and middle phase of their perimenopause. By the time they reach sixty to sixty-five years of age, the flushes and sweats are usually much, much better.

The thing is, for many women the other problems associated with perimenopause only really start to kick in when the hormone levels become low or non-existent. Symptoms like vaginal pain and irritation, bladder infections, bladder irritations, urinary tract infections (UTIs) can start anytime during the perimenopause, but they tend to really get intense when oestrogen levels fall away to nothing.

Sadly, unlike other symptoms of the perimenopause, problems related to low oestrogen, such as vaginal issues, usually don't get better by themselves and can worsen the longer you live. I have to be honest, whenever I meet a woman with menopause-related vaginal symptoms I always warn her that these problems will probably never go away completely, that she will possibly need some kind of treatment to keep her quality of life and health improved for the rest of her days. When I prescribe vaginal oestrogen, creams or pessaries, I normally write 'Forever' on the file. Take note – the leaflet that comes with a box of vaginal oestrogen usually says *Take the lowest dose for the shortest amount of time* on it. Completely counter-intuitive!

That might sound a bit shocking, but the important thing is that the help is available and if you need it forever, you get it forever. (See Chapters 4 and 5 for a full discussion of the vagina and menopause.)

How you know you're out the other side of menopause

So those are the sorts of symptoms that will let you know that you're in perimenopause or menopause, but what about symptoms of post-menopause? Well, obviously the big one is that you no longer have a menstrual cycle. If you've had experience of the symptoms of peri-menopause and then your periods stopped and haven't restarted within twelve months, you know that you are now post-menopausal. The ovaries have retired and are off sunning themselves in Barbados, all their hard work over!

This means you are reproductively done. For some women, this makes them feel relieved – goodbye contraception, goodbye heavy bleeding, and bring on the white trousers already. Other women feel like something has been lost or taken from them and instead of feeling liberated, they feel redundant. Lots of emotions can be swirling around inside you when you say farewell to your monthly bleeds and your fertility.

I have mentioned bleeding in post-menopausal women before, but I'm going to keep repeating it because it's a very important point. For doctors, nurses, gynaecologists and their patients, one of the most worrying symptoms in an older woman is post-menopausal bleeding. If your periods are finished and you haven't seen a natural cycle in months or years, we assume your fertility is gone, your ovaries are asleep, and we expect your ovary hormone levels will be quite low. This is most likely to be a permanent situation if you are over fifty; you stop seeing menstrual bleeds, and that's the end of it.

But if, all of a sudden, you get a return of vaginal bleeding and you are over fifty and you haven't bled for a few years, that can be a warning sign – it's a red flag symptom of womb-lining cancer. If this occurs, you need to get it checked out immediately. It could be something else entirely, but your GP, and often a gynaecologist, needs to find out what's causing it and hopefully eliminate the scary causes. When your body has shut down the reproductive cycle, you should not experience vaginal bleeding. This is no problem during perimenopause, no problem if you have intermittent and unpredictable bleeding – that comes with the territory of the transition. But once you have stopped bleeding for twelve to twenty-four months and you are over fifty, that should be that and it shouldn't happen again. If it does occur, treat it seriously and get it checked out.

When it comes to menopause symptoms, at whatever stage you're at, there is help to manage them and you have options. Once you're informed and happy with your choices, that's what matters. Almost no one has to suffer through years of crappy symptoms any more, and we can all be grateful for that.

KEY TAKEAWAYS

- You can start to experience perimenopause at any age, but most of us will notice symptoms kicking off sometime in our forties.

- At that stage the symptoms are very unpredictable and may be severe at times and disappear at other times. You won't be able to predict how it will go for you. And there are NO blood tests to identify this stage of the perimenopause either, so it's easily misdiagnosed.

- The timeline for your symptoms may not be linear – you may have good months and bad months, good years and bad years, but help is always available if you know who to ask.

- As you get closer to fifty, your ovaries are now at retirement age, when they are thinking of packing it in completely. You usually stop getting monthly bleeds around now, but you may still have quite noticeable menopause symptoms – they may even be a little worse, they may not be – again, highly unpredictable. So, if you are on HRT, do not be disappointed to find you need it throughout your fifties. If you are not on HRT and your perimenopause symptoms get worse after your periods stop, go talk to someone!

- By the age of sixty to sixty-five years, many people find their need for hormone support drops off and they often stop their HRT on their own and muddle through the next forty years without too much difficulty. But the decision on if/when to stop taking HRT is up to you.

3. So, am I menopausal?

What you need to know
before going to see your doctor

This is a huge question for so many women because when you look up 'menopause symptoms', you are confronted with a list longer than your arm. It includes all sorts of things that could be menopause-related but could be something else entirely. This makes it difficult to arrive at a definite diagnosis at times, and GPs and health care practitioners can make mistakes. I miss the diagnosis myself from time to time and it is my speciality! An added problem is that GPs and primary care teams are working under unprecedented pressure. (Doctors are leaving the profession in great numbers, heading to other English-speaking countries where they can make a good living and have a better work-life balance.) It's a perfect storm: you've got a difficult diagnosis to make, one that requires patience and careful listening and discussion, and you've got overworked, under-pressure doctors who have a clock ticking loudly all the while and a line of patients outside the door.

I've heard women complain of this so often, either feeling they aren't listened to at all, or else they are listened to but everything is put down to that handy catch-all term 'menopause'. Or else it's not, and they are diagnosed with depression and offered anti-depressants. It can be a challenge to find a good doctor who knows their climacteric from their elbow and who can guide you successfully and confidently through this transition period. Even if you are fortunate to have a sympathetic GP who understands peri/menopause, it may be hard for them to unravel your story. This means that the more information you have gathered yourself, the better. You can be your own best advocate, if that's necessary.

This is the big health warning with this chapter: you may suspect you are perimenopausal, the guidelines may support your suspicion, you may feel it is the right time for you to try HRT, but that does not mean your GP will necessarily agree with you or have the time, or indeed the skill, to discuss all the treatment options with you. You need to do a bit of homework first, so that you're able to conduct the conversation you need to have with your GP.

As we saw in the last chapter, perimenopause is a minefield of symptoms – days without symptoms, odd symptoms, some bleeding, lots of bleeding, no bleeding. It can take on so many forms, and no two women are exactly the same. That's a diagnostic nightmare for any doctor. It's also a nightmare for the woman experiencing it, because you're never quite sure of what you're feeling, you doubt yourself, wondering if it is menopause-related or you're dismissing something as 'menopause' when you shouldn't be. For God's sake, I'm a doctor and I wasn't confident enough to recognize my own symptoms as being related to the menopause! So, I get it, believe me. It can feel so lonely in perimenopause world because you constantly feel uncertain about what exactly you're feeling, you're not sure if something is a symptom or a passing figary and if you go to your GP and have a less than satisfactory discussion about it, you end up feeling even more lonely and unable to express what exactly is going on with you.

I know there are plenty of good stories about positive menopause consultations, but it is also the case that I hear a lot of bad stories, some of which leave me angry at times. As this seems to be a relatively common experience, and because this particular story happened as recently as spring 2022, I'm going to share a case that might strike a chord with many of you. I think it highlights some of the key problems you can hit when you seek advice about and treatment for perimenopause symptoms.

The woman in question – let's call her Gill – is fifty years old and is an occupational therapist, so she's used to medical conversations and dealing with fellow medical professionals. Gill first talked to a nurse at her GP practice, describing her symptoms. The nurse urged her to make an appointment with the doctor to request a trial of bio-identical HRT. This is how she describes that experience.

> I made the appointment, then prepared for it by writing down all my symptoms: anxiety, paranoid thinking, low mood, irritability, constant fatigue, feeling overwhelmed, memory loss/brain fog. I also noted that I had osteopenia [bones that are weaker than normal, but not yet into the osteoporosis range]. I read up on HRT on

the British Menopause Society website and also on the Menopause Hub website [www.themenopausehub.ie]. Then, armed with all my research, I went in to talk to my GP.

The GP listened to the symptoms, then she told me that HRT is only evidence-based for the treatment of physical symptoms, such as hot flushes. Therefore, if she were to prescribe it for me, it would not be a valid prescription (or words to that effect). As breast cancer is in my family, she wanted me to see a breast endo-crine specialist/general surgeon first. When I again pointed to the severity of my symptoms, which were affecting my quality of life and also affecting my ability to do my job properly and effectively, she told me that if HRT helped with fatigue, then every woman on the pill would never experience fatigue and would be bouncing with energy because the same hormones are in both medications.

At this stage I felt defeated, as if she had taken my energy – and my confidence along with it. At the end of the consultation, as well as ruling out any further discussion on HRT between us and making it clear she would not prescribe it, she suggested I con-sider taking anti-depressants instead as that would address my mood issues without increasing my risk of breast cancer. I appreciated her concern regarding cancer risk, but that suggestion made me feel like my experience of the symptoms was being reduced, dismissed. I left the clinic feeling very low and out of options. It wasn't what I needed at all.

Now, this infuriates me because while the GP was right to assess cancer risk and advise caution, she was incorrect on some points of fact. HRT and the contraceptive pill do not contain 'the same hormones' – yes, they both contain the hormones oestrogen and progestagen, but the doses and molecules are completely different. HRT is a tiny sup-plemental dose of the female hormones that are *already in your blood right now*, and HRT just adds them in a steady, balancing dose. In truth, it's safe to prescribe HRT for nearly everyone. The pill, on the other hand, is a sledgehammer dose of oestrogen and progestagen that is used to supress follicle development in the ovaries and prevent preg-nancy. Comparing both medications is a chalk and cheese situation, and I'm surprised that a GP would not know this.

Those answers did not adequately address the patient's questions. And if a medical person like Gill can feel defeated by this sort of conversation, what about the completely non-medical person who feels unable or ill-equipped to argue the case? You can see how quickly things can go wrong and what could be a positive consultation ends up feeling negative – which is a loss for both doctor and patient because neither of them wants that. Moreover, the NICE guidelines on menopause and HRT specifically advise doctors not to offer antidepressants as a first-line medication for menopause-related mood disorder. So, in this case, that GP either did not know the rules or misinterpreted them.

The low-tech reality of diagnosing the onset of menopause

So, what does happen when you go to your GP complaining of headaches or anxiety or brain fog or heavy periods or insomnia or . . . any of the myriad pain-in-the-ass symptoms that might just characterize the reality that your reproductive system is on the wane? Okay, I would suggest that, before you even make the appointment, you email your GP clinic and ask if they follow the NICE guidelines on menopause.* If they say, 'Huh?', go somewhere else.

The first thing to know is that there is no blood test readily available to you or your GP to assist in the diagnosis of the perimenopause. This is a myth that has somehow taken hold, and women often turn up at their GP or menopause clinic asking for a blood test so that they'll 'know if it's menopause for real'. A simple, straightforward blood test that delivers an accurate diagnosis does not exist. Yes, there is a blood test that could, theoretically, *suggest* perimenopause (for example, testing levels of hormones made in the ovary that decline as menopause approaches), but it is not very reliable and therefore a waste of your

* The National Institute for Health and Care Excellence is a UK-based organization that develops evidence-based recommendations to improve health and social care. We don't have an equivalent in Ireland, so Irish doctors regularly refer to UK guidance.

money – and it costs a lot of money at that. Similarly, if you've heard that there is saliva testing that can diagnose perimenopause, that's garbage and do not pay for such a thing. As with the blood test, yes, there is a saliva test that's available, but it is not considered reliable.

The other test that is available is to measure the reproductive hormone FSH – follicle stimulating hormone. We met this hormone in Chapter 1, along with its close cousins, luteinizing hormone (LH), estradiol and progesterone. FSH is generated by the pituitary gland in the brain and is essential for the healthy functioning of the ovaries. It can be very useful to measure FSH in the blood, but there is a proviso: FSH, estradiol and progesterone are notoriously fluctuant and do not always reflect the hour-to-hour, day-to-day variation that occurs during the perimenopause. This is another reason why a clinical diagnosis is preferred. However, we do use sex hormone blood testing in some circumstances – mainly for women under forty years of age suspected of premature ovarian insufficiency (POI, see Chapter 6). We also occasionally use it for women over fifty years of age to help identify the end of contraceptive need.

So, what can your FSH levels tell us? We take a blood sample and from that we can determine the level of FSH. If your level is high, and you are under forty, that could indicate premature ovarian insufficiency (POI), polycystic ovary syndrome (PCOS), ovarian tumour, Turner Syndrome (see Chapter 6), or perimenopause. If your FSH level is low, that could indicate a problem with ovary function, a problem with pituitary gland function, a problem with hypothalamus function, or that you are severely underweight. So in among those various possibilities, you can see that perimenopause could be detected and confirmed by a FSH test.

For us health-care providers, the protocol for using the FSH test is as follows. If you come to us as a patient and you haven't had a period in over a year, and *only* if you ask us to do so in order to know when you can stop using contraception, we can offer to measure your FSH level in order to confirm that you are post-menopausal. You can picture FSH like a mother trying to wake her kids up for school. At the beginning of your normal menstrual cycle, FSH comes roaring out of your anterior pituitary gland and is hell-bent on shaking up your egg follicles. When the eggs respond as they should do ('I'm up already!'), the FSH levels drop down again. Her job is done, time to get a coffee, walk the dog, go to work. But if the eggs are exhausted, they do not respond to FSH as they are meant to – so she yells even louder. This makes your FSH levels climb even higher in the desperate hope that those lazy eggs will start to wake up and get organized again. But if you're over fifty years of age, chances are they won't.

If you are over fifty and your FSH is measuring over 30 IU/L (international units per litre), those eggs are likely never waking up again. (*FSH, sister, you are wasting your time!*) There will be no more pregnancies and no more periods and those FSH levels will remain at a high level throughout your post-reproductive years. So, if you feel you are post-menopausal – and you come to us to confirm that – your age, the fact of no longer menstruating and a high level of FSH will together tell us that this diagnosis is correct.

So now you're thinking, *But why can't you just test my FSH in order to tell me I'm perimenopausal?* From a practical point of view, we do not routinely measure FSH unless we need to because it's seen as a waste of taxpayer money. Yes, FSH has a big role in gynae diagnosis, but diagnosing symptoms of perimenopause is not one of them. And it's not just about money and the expense of the test. There's also the fact that you can have classic menopause symptoms, and very much need HRT or other menopause therapies, but have a low level of FSH, or you can be symptom-free and not interested in HRT and have an elevated level of FSH. Many women experience perimenopausal symptoms long before their final menstrual period, so it is not uncommon for women to still be having menstrual cycles and normal FSH levels while actively going through perimenopause. The one does not exclude the other. The problem is that, as with all things hormonal, there are fluctuations and anomalies, and that makes the tests less reliable for diagnoses like menopause.

After all that, I have to tell you that the answer to diagnosing if you're perimenopausal is extremely low tech. We diagnose perimenopause by listening to you carefully, recognizing the link between your age and your symptoms, and then saying, 'I think you may be in the perimenopause.' That's it. We can eliminate other potential causes, such as cancer, thyroid and adrenal disease, et cetera, and then we are left with the logical explanation – logical because of your age – that the process of winding down the menstrual cycle has indeed begun for you.

Doing your homework to find the right GP

So, how do you go about getting the support and management help you need when you are experiencing symptoms? There's no easy answer here, I'm afraid, because every patient is different and every doctor is different, too. I've honestly heard so many horror stories from women who came out of their GP clinic in tears, left with a feeling of not knowing where to turn next. That's a really tough situation and, to be blunt, I can't save you from it. I can give you tips on reading up on menopause, having the vocabulary down, bringing your list of symptoms and questions with you – but that doesn't guarantee you get a sympathetic or menopause-knowledgeable doctor. It's hit and miss, that's just how it is.

But what I will say on this is that it is slowly changing. For example, Dr Brian Kennedy, a colleague of mine, a menopause guru and just an amazing Tipperary GP, set up a Telegram group for menopause discussion among doctors – so we can sound each other out, ask for advice, update each other on new studies and medications. To his astonishment – and mine – that group has now grown to include over 800 medics, all eager to learn about the menopause and to try to do right by their patients. Now that's progress! It shows me that the desire to learn is there, and that it is growing all the time.

What you have to remember as well is that the menopause remains under-resourced in Irish medicine. In the UK there are hormone gynaecologists, but the Republic of Ireland is lagging in this regard. There are no hormone gynaecologists in Ireland dedicated specifically to menopause, PMS, et cetera, and there are very few services, which means the services that are there are struggling to keep pace with demand. There are a few private menopause clinics that you can access yourself, without needing a referral, but only now are we getting hospital-based dedicated menopause services.

GPs are left dealing with this shortfall in services. As doctors, we don't have much training on menopause at medical college; a lot of

GPs feel a bit out of their depth when a woman comes in with a list of random symptoms and major anxiety to go along with it. They may not be sure what to do – and they don't want to do something wrong, of course. There aren't enough GPs and practices to cope with demand, so your GP is likely doing their best but under difficult circumstances. You can't accept poor service or a crappy attitude, but you can be understanding and try to meet them halfway as much as possible.

That means doing your homework – like you're doing right now by reading this book. Try emailing your existing GP surgery and asking about making a menopause appointment – ask do they have a GP in the surgery with menopause experience and make sure your appointment is with that person. If they do not respond or if they do not have any interest in menopause care, shop around – assuming you have the money and patience to do that.

Think about what you're experiencing, and gather the knowledge. Make a diary of your symptoms – focus on the worst three, for starters, and we can eventually move down the list – keep a period diary, whether it's a red X on your wall calendar or a period tracker app, and bring this information along with you to the discussion.

You have to keep an open mind about what the symptoms might be telling you. It might be perimenopause; it might not be. Follow the evidence, as the TV detectives say. Try to use the correct vocabulary, so there are no annoying misunderstandings. And write down what they say, so you can go back over it afterwards, make sure it makes sense to you and that you agree with it.

What I would say to you, and to GPs, is that if you are of a certain age and you believe you might be perimenopausal, you probably are. Classic menopause symptoms in a healthy patient aged between forty and fifty probably mean . . . you guessed it . . . menopause! And we are finding that many women arrive into the surgery for a consultation having already diagnosed themselves – and they are almost always correct. And you do not need a rake of blood tests to confirm this and start taking action.

KEY TAKEAWAYS

- There is no readily available blood test that will accurately diagnose perimenopause – if you think you are in it, chances are you are right!

- There is no saliva test that will diagnose perimenopause.

- Your doctor should make the diagnosis of perimenopause by listening to you and recognizing the symptoms – unless you come under special circumstances, such as POI (see Chapter 6).

- When we experience emotional or mental symptoms, it comes easily to us to look for external causes. I did it myself – when I had menopause symptoms. That's how I ended up on anti-depressants when what I really needed was HRT. A sudden mood disorder in a middle-aged woman presenting with one or more symptoms of perimenopause is less likely to be reactive depression and more likely to be perimenopause and hormonal imbalance.

- You can get a blood test diagnosis of 'post-menopause' if you are over fifty and have gone one year without natural periods. You don't need to do this test to try HRT.

- Do your research, read up on menopause online and in books, write down your symptoms, and know what you want before you go to see your GP. You can ask for what you want. If your GP refuses your request, ask them to explain their reasons for doing so, including the guidelines that are informing their decision.

4. What the heck is happening to my vagina?

This is the question I hear very often at my clinic: *What the heck is happening to my vagina?* The focus can be so much on hot flushes and brain fog and those sorts of menopause symptoms that women can forget the entire show is being staged in the womb, ovaries, cervix and vagina. So, when things begin to change for them 'down there', it can come as a bit of a shock and cause a lot of consternation and sometimes confusion. In this chapter we're going to have a very direct look at your vagina, its anatomy, how the hormones affect it, and how the change in hormones and hormonal loss affect it. This is a crucial discussion because, as we saw in Chapter 2, when it comes to vaginal health problems, the symptoms typically do not get better on their own.

Your vagina and beyond – a refresher course

Not everyone is familiar with their own anatomy. Some people struggle to give the correct names to the different parts of the body that are connected to having periods, having sex, having babies and such. It is worth spending a few minutes making sure we are all using the same names for the areas of our bodies that we need to be aware of (and talk about) throughout our lives.

All the stuff that is encased in your pelvic area is known as the genito-urinary system – *genito* meaning genitals and sexual/reproductive equipment, and *urinary* for the peeing-related equipment: the bladder, urethra (the tube you pee through) and the 'opening' or meatus.

Your vagina, your womb, the cervix, the fallopian tubes, the ovaries and the ligaments and the muscles that support them – all of these structures fit in the pelvis. They mostly sit on top of a large, trampoline-shaped strappy muscle called the *pelvic floor*. All of this is

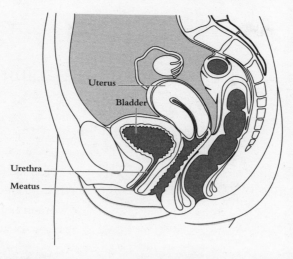

Uterus

Bladder

Urethra

Meatus

Figure 1: Your genito-urinary system covers everything in your pelvis, from vulva to bladder

designed for pregnancy and childbirth, that's its ultimate purpose, and it must be ready to perform that function.

Looking more closely at what makes up the GU system

Starting from the outside in, as it were, let's begin with the *vulva*. The outer surface of your genital area is called the vulva. This is an umbrella term for all the external genitalia and it includes: the mons pubis, which is the chubby bit above your vulva that is meant to have hair on it, the labia majora and the labia minora, which we call the lips; and your clitoris, which hides under a little hood of skin above where your pee comes out. This is an area of dense sensory tissue and is ground zero for most women in terms of sexual arousal.

There are two different sets of lips or *labia* : the bigger, outside ones where your pubic hair grows (labia majora) and the smaller, inner ones where hair doesn't grow (labia minora). The vaginal opening is in between the inner lips.

To the back, behind the opening of the *vagina* and towards the opening that is your anus, that bit of stretchy skin is called the *perineum*. If you were ever pregnant or gave birth, you'll have heard about your perineum *a lot*.

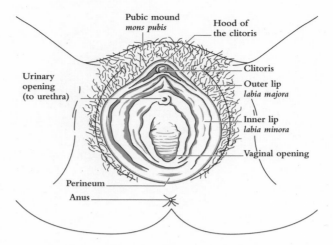

Figure 2: This is a doctor's eye view of your beautiful, hard-working vagina

To the front of the vaginal opening you have your urethral opening, the *meatus*, and this is where you release urine from. Your clitoris sits above the urethral meatus. This whole area has an abundant supply of sensory nerve endings and is known as an 'erogenous zone'. The clitoris is usually a highly sensitive erogenous area, although this varies a lot from woman to woman. Some women are more sensitive to sexual arousal inside the vagina, some around the clitoris, while some are aroused by non-genital stimuli (for example, touching the breasts).

Going inside, where you usually cannot see, you have all your reproductive structures. We usually have to use a plastic or metal device called a 'speculum' to see inside the vagina and up to the *cervix*. Deeper still, you have the womb, the tubes and the ovaries.

The vagina

The vagina is an amazingly crafted bit of biological engineering that acts as a passageway from the outside world through to the inner depths of the womb, which in turn connects through to the tubes and into the pelvis beyond. The vagina is particularly geared up for childbirth, with walls that are very convoluted. Convoluted literally means 'in folds' – the walls of the vagina are like one of those paper fans you made in school, with all the folds sitting on top of each other. The

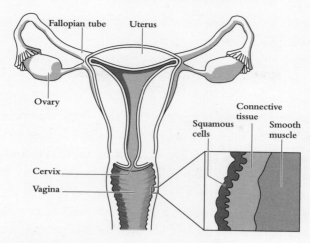

Figure 3: Your womb requires a good hormonal balance to do its work

folds and ridges are called *rugae*, which is Latin for wrinkles or folds, and that is what you find in an oestrogen-rich vagina – lots of folds of tissue. They can stretch and expand, but then bounce back to (mostly) how they were before. When you are in the later stages of pregnancy, other hormones are released to make the walls of your vagina even more soft and stretchy, so it's certainly not just a straight, flat tube like a lot of people see when you draw a picture of it.

The womb and its cervix

The beautiful, soft, pink, squishy, pear-shaped box inside your pelvis, where your period blood comes down from and where little humans are carried, is called the womb or the *uterus*. At the bottom of the uterus there's a kind of narrow passageway and this is the cervix (from the Latin for the neck, of the uterus).

This passageway is part of the womb, but it actually sits up in the deepest part of the vagina – you can feel it if you put your finger inside your vagina. The cervix has many jobs, but it primarily acts as a security gate so that stuff from outside the vagina can't get deep inside. Interestingly, the inside of the womb is sterile. No air gets up there because inside the cervical canal is a wad of special mucus that has protective properties. However, the cells on the outside of the cervix are susceptible to viral cancers, which is why we get smear tests done for HPV-related cell changes that can lead to cancers.

The tubes

Leading off the 'box' of the womb are tiny little channels, one on the left and one on the right, and these are the fallopian tubes. They are the passageways for eggs (ova) travelling from each ovary down into the womb, as well as the route by which sperms get to those eggs. When you have a period, the blood and tissue travel down the cervical canal, into the vagina, and emerge through the vaginal opening, called the *interoitus*. The area on the outside, around the opening, is called the vulva, which is the umbrella term for all the external genitalia.

The bladder, urethra and meatus

Urine is passed outside the body via the urethral meatus. If you looked at your meatus with a mirror, it ought to look small and tight and blush-pink in colour, regardless of your skin colour. Below the urethra is the part of the vulva where the vaginal opening is, and that whole part of you is called 'the vestibule'. At the vaginal opening are a few mucus-secreting glands that are usually too small to see but that are helpful in keeping the vestibule moist and pH-balanced. But God help you if those openings get blocked up! You can get an abscess (which is not uncommon, especially in younger women) and they are *painful* and require immediate attention.

What happens in the vulva and vagina during menopause

Oestrogen and other sex hormones are necessary for many different functions, but their loss can be really noticed when it comes to having a healthy vagina and vulva. Oestrogen is one hard-working hormone and when it quits, it has a serious effect. During perimenopause, changes in the tissues that make up the vagina, the vulva, the bladder, the urethra and the pelvic floor are common, but are not always talked about — and not always asked about at a medical check-up, by either doctor or patient.

All the tissue and all the organs in your pelvis – the vagina and vulva, the urethra and bladder and the whole pelvic floor muscle mass – come from the same part of the human embryo and are replete with oestrogen and other sex hormone receptors. The more oestrogen you have available to you during puberty, the thicker and healthier the vulva, vagina and other pelvic organs can become.

If you looked at your vulva, you might start to notice changes as you approached your last period. You might have less pubic hair (if you haven't Brazilianed it all away). The tissues can become less of a blush-pink and more of a pale yellow. You might even see little red dots, called *petechiae*, on the vulva from damaged blood vessels. If you were able to see the inner tissues of the vagina, like I can when I use the speculum, you would notice that they too are becoming paler and somewhat dry and that the rugae, those nooks and crannies, are starting to disappear. Over time, the lips themselves, the labia majora and labia minora, tend to shrivel up a little, getting smaller and less stretchy, or they may disappear altogether, as we sometimes see with the small inner lips. The outer lips might even stick together up at the top, near your clitoris, while the clitoris itself can shrivel up slightly and the sensitive patch of skin above it – the clitoral hood – may disappear. Oh, what joy is aging!

In addition to the changes arising from menopause, as we age the blood supply to the vagina – in fact to all of our pelvic organs – drops off a bit. So whatever little oestrogen is left in the blood can't even get down to the vagina walls. The loss of oestrogen as menopause progresses can have a big effect. There is a special name for all this: genito-urinary syndrome of menopause, or GSM. Now, some people are not overly bothered by vulval or vaginal symptoms, but other people really struggle with them. Let's work our way through the various aspects of GSM.

All the tissues of the body are made up of cells and extra-cellular components of tissue (the stuff outside the cells). Two such components are proteins the body makes to keep tissues strong and elastic – collagen and elastin. Collagen and elastin levels naturally fall with age, but for us women, oestrogen loss also contributes to the process. You'll notice the decline in collagen and elastin in your skin, and this may help you to imagine what's happening on the inside. Skin loses its plumpness, becomes saggy and does not bounce back as it once did. Since I got older – I'm in my sixties now – I notice that my cheek skin (*on my face!*) blows around like a sheet on the line when I am using the hair dryer. And in the ladies' room, when I put my hands under the dryer, the skin blows all over the place. It's kind of gross, but it's a natural part of aging. I don't particularly love it, but I try to see it as part of the privilege of growing older.

The body uses collagen to make connective tissues, so the decline in collagen reduces the elasticity of the vagina and the vulva. Elastin breakdown similarly affects the stretchiness of the vagina and vulva. Elastin is a stretchy, tough protein with a long shelf life and we rely on it for the stretchability of our heart and joints and lots of other tissues that move (this may be in part why heart disease seems to be prevented by HRT use in later life – see Chapter 17).

As well as collagen and elastin, the vagina walls rely on lots of mucus production from the glands in the deeper part of the vagina, near the cervix. As we enter the menopause, however, many women notice that the moisture that normally comes down from the vagina starts to become less abundant. If you are in charge of laundry in a house with younger women and you come across a pile of clothes on the floor, believe you me, you know straight away which knickers have been worn and which haven't. But with older women, our natural vaginal secretions dry up and very little material comes down out of our vagina any more. This saves on laundry but has unfortunate potential consequences – our natural vaginal lubrication becomes less profuse, scantier, and we might feel dry and prone to irritation.

A shift in the mucosal tissue as well as a reduction in good bacteria (lactobacilli) can cause an increase in the normal acidic pH of the vagina. The pH is a number that describes the acidity or alkalinity of a tissue or liquid. The vagina has a healthy pH level that needs to be maintained: a PH of 7 is neutral or midway, 1 is highly acidic and 14 is highly alkaline. The vagina has a team of bacteria, led by the predominant lactobacilli, that live in there and keep harmful germs away. The lactobacilli bacteria make by-products that are acidic, so a healthy vagina, replete with lactobacilli, should have a pH of around

4–5. On the acidic side. If the numbers of lactobacilli go down – stress and antibiotics being the most common causes of reduction in lactobacilli numbers, the pH goes up, and this can cause vaginal odour and irritations, like burning and itch. It can also allow for the growth of less helpful vaginal bacteria, such as gardnerella, which in turn can lead to the very common vaginal irritation condition known as BV (bacterial vaginosis).

Another relatively common set of GSM symptoms are to do with urination: lots can go awry with the 'waterworks', such as urine leakage, having to pee too often, burning when you pee, bladder or urinary tract infections (UTIs) and repeated thrush infections. At any time, women are more at risk of UTIs than men. That's because our urethra is so short, so it is easier for unhealthy bacteria to make their way from the outside to the inside. Also, our vagina and anus, which can be a source of bacteria, are geographically close to our urethra – unlike the penis opening, which is miles away (well, actually centimetres) from the back passage.

As the urethral opening is impacted by oestrogen loss in the menopause, it starts to gape a bit, which can lead to 'urethral meatus dilation'. This makes it even easier to have bacteria stroll inside, so you can end up with repeat UTIs. This is why many elderly women get recurrent infections, even more likely if you have to wear a continence pad or an adult nappy. Some small studies have shown that elderly ladies in care homes might be protected against recurrent bladder infections by using some low-dose oestrogen cream to the urethral area.

The weight of the womb is carried by the big trampoline-shaped muscle called the pelvic diaphragm – or pelvic floor. It becomes weaker in the absence of oestrogen and with aging, which presents the possibility of the womb dropping a little in the pelvis in what is known as 'prolapse'. This can become more of a problem during the menopause when the sensation of 'something coming down' through the vagina is more common. A severe version of prolapse – known as a 'procidentia' – is when the womb drops so far down into the vagina it is actually hanging outside of the body, like a big pink aubergine between your legs.

The worst case of procidentia I ever saw was in an 85-year-old woman, who was the living embodiment of that old attitude of keeping things silent and hidden. This was back in the 1980s, when I was training in the Mater Hospital, and this lady was on the gynae ward for a hysterectomy. I was told to get her details for the chart. She was a lovely, cheerful woman who entertained my medical student awkwardness with good humour. I started with the despicable 'What brought you into hospital?' and she whipped back the blanket on her bed to reveal a procidentia.

'Jesus!' I said (always the professional) and she laughed. 'How long have you been like this?' I asked.

She said it had been about thirty years, but now she needed to get it fixed because it was preventing her from riding her bicycle. My queen! I will never forget that brave lady. But how she had lived with it for thirty years, I do not know. Everything abraded it, snagged it, everything must have caused pain, and she had regular bleeding as a result of the trauma that just going about her day caused to it. And she only came in for help when she couldn't cycle so far any more.

Now, let's talk about sex

As you may well imagine, all of these changes can have a big impact on your sex life. The walls of the vagina are meant to be self-lubricating. Their stretchy nature, and the natural moisture that is created in the vagina, offer a 'glide surface' when you're having penetrative sex or doing vigorous exercise or whenever there is activity inside the vagina. When your collagen and elastin are undermined and your mucus production declines, you will lose that glide surface. In extreme cases, you can be unlucky enough to end up with what's called 'vaginal atrophy'. This is where the walls of the vagina are so thin that they can become scratched and abraded and rough and then start to rub off each other in a sore way. Some women have told me it's like two pieces of sandpaper rubbing off each other, just to give you an image that will remain burned into your mind's eye forever!

Oestrogen loss may lead to thinner, drier and smaller pelvic structures. Your mons gets flatter and stores less fat, so it's no longer a nice cushion when someone else's pubic bone is pushing against yours. As we've seen, your labia can shrink and shrivel and sometimes disappear altogether. Worse yet, the lips can fuse together, blocking the opening to your vagina. Your clitoral hood can shrink back, and you might find you get an irritation from your clothing rubbing against your now unprotected sensitive spot.

All of this can make penetrative sex very, very uncomfortable where before it had been enjoyable. Sex drive can already be taking a hit during perimenopause because our waning levels of another joyous female hormone – testosterone – can reduce sexual desire (I talk about this in Chapters 9 and 12). But even in the presence of a good libido, a dry, painful vulva and/or vagina will be an enormous barrier to a satisfying sex life. Painful sex, called 'dyspareunia', is said to affect almost half of all menopausal patients, but fewer than 25 per cent seek help, which is heartbreaking when you consider what they might be going through in their daily lives.

Vaginal atrophy is an awful situation. I've had patients who were so desperately unwell that during sex they actually scraped and scratched themselves internally to the point where, as the tissues of the vagina started to heal, they merged into each other, and the two sides and the front and back of the vagina actually started to stick to one other. In other words, the vagina was closing over in a condition known as vaginal wall fusion. If the vaginal walls become adherent, you can imagine the pain that might occur if you tried to walk or sit down or, God forbid, have penetrative sex. Those two surfaces that were stuck together would rip apart and you would have bleeding and pain. It's a distressing thought – but the key is not to let it get that far. There is help for this, and you have to go seek it out.

I remember a lady who came in for a menopause consult. She was maybe sixty-five and she told me that she found sex painful, and it often caused bleeding. She also complained of pain when walking upstairs or getting up from a low chair, so I figured this wasn't your usual vaginal dryness. We needed to talk and I needed to examine her.

When I looked, the outside of her vagina – the whole vulval area – was a yellow colour, with lots of little broken blood vessels all over it. The labia, or lips, had all but disappeared and I could only make out the smallest of vaginal openings. She had had several vaginal birth deliveries, so this made no sense.

I used loads of K Y Jelly for lubrication and tried to pass the tip of

my finger into her vagina. She yelped at my touch, and I realized that
the walls of her vagina had completely fused together. I could not
believe this woman was having penetrative sex. I asked her how long
she had been like this, and she said for about ten years. She had asked
her GP if she could get some HRT for this and was told, 'No, that
gives you breast cancer.' I could have cried.

We started on what was quite a long journey, which began with the
permission to say no to penetrative sex. She used lashings of local oestrogen cream and made a few trips to the gynae physio. She did really
well once she got that help, but I was deeply affected by that case and
by what some people put up with. I have heard that most women with
incontinence – leaking urine, or sometimes faeces, when they cough,
laugh or see a toilet – wait over five years before asking for help. I
know I keep saying this, but it really is heartbreaking.

The severity of the effect of oestrogen loss on sex varies from
woman to woman. Some will find that it's simply too painful to have
sex at all, while other women will find that they can participate in sex
but don't get arousal to the same extent, which can be very upsetting.
It's no surprise, then, that some women's attitudes towards sex undergo
a change in the menopause. You might not want to have penetrative
vaginal sex. This might be due to painful soreness, which naturally is
a big turn-off, or to dryness that robs you of the pleasure you once
enjoyed, or to the fact that your clitoris isn't working like it once did
and that also puts you off.

Lots of women who are relatively easily aroused and very capable of
successful orgasm find this starts to change in the menopause. Becoming stimulated and then eventually reaching orgasm can become more
difficult and can take longer. Stemming from that, you might be getting a whole load of sexual friction as you try to achieve orgasm, and
then you're getting sore from that. Add to this tiredness and disturbed
sleep patterns and, really, the whole thing just becomes a big old chore.
You can end up feeling that even if you are motivated to have sex or
masturbate, the effort to become aroused and then to orgasm becomes
too tiresome. This is understandable, but it's also really sad because sex
and masturbation are such a fun part of a healthy life. And it can, of
course, have an adverse effect on your intimate relationships.

Vaginal atrophy has been a neglected issue in women's health. The

European REVIVE Survey 2016, involving participants from Italy, Germany, Spain and the UK, concluded that uro-genital atrophy is an under-recognized, under-diagnosed and thus under-treated condition. It recommended a public awareness campaign, with a focus on educating women about the symptoms and also on educating gynaecologists, urologists, dermatologists, general practitioners, sexual health clinicians, specialist nurses and practice nurses. The more awareness, the better for those trying to live with these silent, hidden conditions. I truly hope the days of suffering in silence are at an end.

Don't panic!

This whole smorgasbord of horror is GSM, and we are all going to be affected by some of it at some stage, I hate to tell you. But while all of this may sound alarming, do try not to panic: most women do not have extreme symptoms of GSM, but just a little bit of dryness and possibly some loss of comfort during sex or masturbation or examinations. And, crucially, there are ways of treating and managing symptoms. In the next chapter, I'll go through them.

KEY TAKEAWAYS

- Vaginal dryness and genito-urinary problems are very common in menopause, and they don't tend to get better with time, unlike other menopause symptoms.
- It is crucial that you get help and advice, as there is loads we can offer to help you. Read on!

5. The good news – you don't have to put up with vaginal symptoms

Okay, time for the good news. For the most part, the symptoms of GSM can all be helped. You don't have to, and you absolutely should not, put up with them. There is zero value in soldiering through vaginal symptoms because, unlike some of the other menopause problems, like flushes and sweats, vaginal and vulval symptoms tend to get worse as you get older.

Another reason to seek help for these symptoms is to rule out other causes since they can occasionally be a sign of more serious problems. Sometimes, vulvo-vaginal changes in menopause can be a warning sign. There are some pre-cancerous and cancerous conditions of the vulva and vagina that start off with some of the symptoms mentioned in Chapter 4. Getting advice and being examined for persistent problems is essential. Early diagnosis can be key to curing or managing these conditions, but only your GP or a gynaecologist will know how to diagnose the more worrisome issues that can arise.

Having confirmed that your symptoms do arise from menopausal changes, the first thing to think of is the simple ways you can promote the health of your own vagina. There's plenty you can do to protect and maintain the health of your vagina outside of a doctor's office.

Caring for your vagina

Your vagina walls are self-cleaning so there is no need for you to put soap or water or other products up inside your vagina. The natural vaginal mucus has antiseptic properties. You can wash away the secretions from the vulva and the lips and the back passage and the urethra, but the inside of the vagina itself should be left alone. This advice is universal and includes young women, middle-aged women and older women.

When it comes to washing the outer areas, you want to minimize the amount of chemical products that come into contact with your vulva. A mild soap, even one of those over-the-counter, pH-adjusted 'intimate cleansing creams', would be preferable to a big old bar of carbolic. Think gentle – and avoid anything with *parfum* in the ingredients list. And the other thing is that you really don't need to wash it all that often. I've had many patients over the years who thought vaginal irritations could be scrubbed away, but nothing could be further from the truth. In fact, often the more you wash the vagina, the worse the symptoms become as those tissues do not respond well to being scrubbed. They want and need to be left alone as much as possible. What often happens is that if you have a sore vulva or vagina, you get some relief from sitting in a warm tub or having a warm shower because the heat neutralizes the pain, but the washing itself is just going to make the symptoms worse – and it's not therapeutic, for the most part.

Helpful moisturizers and lubricants

There is a range of vaginal moisturizing products that you can buy without a prescription that can really make a big difference to vaginal changes in the menopause. These are specially designed for use inside the vagina and often have a seaweed component, are pH-adjusted and can give long-term relief from the symptoms of dryness – as long as they're not too severe. There are some Irish-made options available, like the KORA products such as Regelle. If you find it awkward to have some young salesperson walking you through all the lovely vaginal moisturizing products – and I wouldn't blame you – you can purchase these products online, if that suits you better.

The same companies that make vaginal moisturizers often do a range of sexual lubricants (lube) as well. I like to use the moisturizer once or twice a week, if not more often, then you can just use the lube when you are engaging in sexual activity. Some are petroleum-based, and others are water-based, and some will suit one person but not another. It's a matter of trial and error to find the best one for you.

One good range is YES organic intimacy products. They can be found in some pharmacies, and online they have a huge range of products, some of which are very entertaining. They do a range for people who enjoy anal sex called YES BUT! The testimonials on their website certainly support the efficacy of their products.

Speaking of anal, over the last few years, I have been really struck by how many older women tell me they don't need contraception because they only have anal sex these days. I have spent a lot of my working life asking people about what they get up to in their intimate encounters – mainly so I know which end of them to take samples from for STI tests! But I can be a bit old school when it comes to the details. I wish I had some people's comfort around discussing sex and sexuality. But I think it's a wonderful development – and it's lovely that people can enjoy each other in so many ways!

The anus is not as stretchy as the vagina (which may be the point, I guess – more sensation) so anal sex is more likely to produce some trauma and bleeding. Also, like everywhere else, the anus becomes a little less moist as you age. So, using lube is really important if you enjoy anal sex. STIs are more readily transmitted via anal sex as there is likely to be a little bit more tissue damage (trauma), so use a condom if you are not in a mutually monogamous relationship. Make sure you use a water or silicone-based lube to avoid damaging the latex in the condom. Let's shoot down one myth: you *can* get pregnant from anal sex. Sperms deposited anywhere near the vagina can and do find their way up inside, so if you are choosing to focus on anal sex, you should still use a condom or be on some form of hormonal contraception.

Oestrogen for the vagina

The ultimate treatment for the symptoms of vaginal oestrogen depletion is to replace the oestrogen locally, right into the vagina and around the vulva, so as to reverse the problem. There are many low-dose products available that do exactly that, including creams, ointments and tiny little pessaries, like pellets or bullet-shaped medicines, that you insert inside the vagina or rub around the outside of the vagina. All such products replenish the oestrogen supplied to those tissues.

Local vaginal hormone use is not the same as HRT in that the hormones do not get into the blood in any meaningful way, therefore the usual cautions and precautions we have for standard HRT use do not apply. Funnily enough, if there is going to be any tiny amount of absorption, it will be when you first start to use the products, i.e. when your vagina is super-thin and dried out. Once those walls thicken up again, thanks to the oestrogen, they act as a barrier to the hormone escaping into the blood. Yet, there has been a little bit of controversy over the safety of using this low-dose vaginal oestrogen to relieve the symptoms of vaginal atrophy in women who would normally be told that they weren't allowed to take HRT. The most common situation we find when this happens is with women who have been diagnosed with breast cancer at some stage in their lives. They often have horrendous vaginal symptoms, either because of the treatments they've received for their breast cancer, or a combination of the treatments and their natural aging. Depending on which oncologist is caring for them, they may either have been quite happily offered vaginal oestrogen or been made to feel terrified about having to use it. Women have reported to me hearing comments such as, 'Well, if you have to, okay, but it will be your own fault if your cancer comes back,' or this type of thing . . . unforgivable, in my book.

There are many observational studies showing that the vaginal oestrogen products allow very little or no systemic absorption of the hormone and that hormone-dependent cancer recurrence rates are not increased by the use of local vaginal oestrogen. However, there has never been a randomized controlled trial (RCT) on breast cancer survivors who were offered vaginal oestrogen, or an identical dummy product, and then followed for between five and ten years to see who did better with regard to breast cancer survivorship – and there probably never will be. This is why the local vaginal oestrogen products will always have written on the boxes *Do not use if you have had breast cancer*, which is so undermining.

Use of vaginal oestrogen for women undergoing breast cancer treatment

There is a small, often quoted study from 2006 regarding the use of vaginal oestrogen by people who are using aromatase inhibitors (AIs) for breast cancer. In this study, they took blood tests to measure the oestrogen levels in patients who were taking AIs as part of their treatment. AIs are used to keep the level of oestrogen in the blood as low as possible (by stopping an enzyme in fat tissue – aromatase – from converting other hormones into oestrogen). The study found that a handful of the women had higher oestrogen blood levels when using vaginal oestrogen.

This study was poor in quality, however. The authors measured the blood levels of oestrogen in only six women on AI therapy. Six! They only used the higher dose Vagifem 25mcg, whereas we only use the 10mcg dose these days. They did not use conventional laboratory methods for measuring blood oestrogen levels – instead they developed a new test themselves because the oestrogen levels were so low, a normal blood test could barely measure them at all. At 14 days they found a rise in oestrogen levels from 3 to 72 pmol/L.* At 28 days that level had dropped back to less than 35 pmol/L, which was reassuring, but they went on to take 'random' samples of blood from the patients and found that two of the ladies had a further increase in oestrogen to 219 pmol/L and 137 pmol/L, respectively. Now, there were other reasons why that might have been happening, for example, when you use high-dose vaginal oestrogen *sporadically*, as opposed to in weekly low doses, more of the hormone can leak into the bloodstream. There was also a suspicion that some of the women in the study had been taking supplements like phytoestrogen, which we know can raise blood oestrogen levels a bit. Who knows?

---

* A *mole* is a unit of measurement used in medical tests and a *picomole* is a fraction of a mole. Modern medical testing is very refined and can pick up minute amounts of a substance in the blood, so results can be given in picomoles per litre (pmol/L). A mole is an amount of a substance that contains a large number (6 followed by 23 zeros) of molecules or atoms. A picomole is one-trillionth of a mole.

Anyway, the word went out: *no vaginal oestrogen for women on A Is*. And so it has been for the last sixteen years. I think it's high time we examine this again, because that study did not find a link between AI and vaginal oestrogen and breast cancer recurrence or spread. But for now, that's the guideline. Although I find that, in Ireland, oncologists' opinions on using vaginal oestrogen with an aromatase inhibitor can be very variable.

Going back to everyone else with a perimenopausal vagina, local oestrogen use is perfectly acceptable even if you have been told to avoid regular HRT. Start by using a good bit of it to get the tissues as healthy as possible and then drop down to the lowest dose that YOU need to keep your vagina feeling good. For as long as you choose to use it.

Professor John Guillebaud is a famous UK gynaecologist who has written a number of definitive books on women's health – and he is still lecturing in his mid-eighties. He has over 300 publications to his credit and his book *Contraception: Your Questions Answered* is my go-to reference for my clinical work. He adores women and women's health and is one of the most engaging lecturers I have ever heard speak. Anyways, Professor Guillebaud once said that if a woman inserted two Vagifem tabs (a brand of pellet-style local oestrogen) into her vagina every week for a year – that is 104 pellets – it would expose her breasts to the same amount of oestrogen as if she swallowed one single oestrogen tablet. That is pretty darn safe, if you ask me.

The downside of local oestrogen treatments is that some vaginal products are expensive. Vaginal oestrogen medication comes in many different types and brands, and some are covered by the Medical Card system in Ireland. There's a cream called Ovestin, a gel called Blissel and the pellets Vagifem or Vagirux. The most recent addition to that menu is a bullet-shaped vaginal pessary called Imvaggis. These are all covered for the most part by the Medical Card system and the Drugs Payment scheme, but they're still not inexpensive – you could be looking at around €20 per month for long-term vaginal oestrogen therapies.

Ospemifene is an oral tablet that is a tissue selective modulator. This means it is designed to improve the function of vaginal oestrogen receptors without affecting the breasts, but is still not recommended after breast cancer. There is an androgen cream called prasterone sold under the trade name Intrarosa which seems to be just as good as oestrogen for vaginal health and should be even 'safer' for women who have vaginal problems but who need to avoid oestrogen as much as possible. Again, it is not yet licensed for use in cases of cancers with oestrogen receptors on them. Neither of these products has a licence for use in Ireland, but both are available in the UK and health-care providers can get them here, no problem, but the cost will be higher as they need to be imported specially.

Local oestrogen treatment – a game-changer for your vaginal well-being

I cannot tell you how life-changing vaginal oestrogen can be. Not only does it improve vaginal comfort and your ability to enjoy sex, but the oestrogen you put in your vagina will also improve the function of the other structures, like your bladder and urethra and, to an extent, your pelvic floor. That means that even symptoms like leaking urine/incontinence and urinary tract infections can get much better with vaginal oestrogen.

It is worth mentioning that if you are going for a pelvic exam or scope and you know that it could be tricky because of lack of elasticity in your vagina, you could ask your doctor to prescribe a vaginal oestrogen cream that you take for a week or two before the exam. That should make the exam easier for you. (These creams are now available over the counter in the UK, so it shouldn't be long before that's the case in Ireland too, and then you'll be able to choose to do this yourself, without the need for a prescription.)

Some women who are already on normal HRT products, like tablets or gels or patches or sprays, will still need local vaginal oestrogen. Even though their blood supply is being replenished with oestrogen, it can struggle to get down to the pelvic floor and the pelvic structures because the blood vessels that carry the oestrogen to those areas might be narrowed. It's very common that you would need both your usual HRT gel/patch or whatever for your other menopausal symptoms, and then have to use vaginal oestrogen as well.

It's important to know that if you have a very dry, sore, sensitive vulva or vagina, anything you apply could cause some problems initially. It's not uncommon for people with a lot of vagina or vulva symptoms to actually feel a little bit more uncomfortable when they first start rubbing in oestrogen cream or inserting oestrogen pellets, but this is a short-lived problem that should improve quite quickly. If it doesn't, you need to go back and talk to your prescribing doctor. It could be that you just need to pull back on the dosage a little bit and let your body get used to the higher level of oestrogen over a longer period of time. Some women notice that when they put oestrogen back into the vagina they get more thrush-type irritation, and that makes sense. Again, this can be improved upon by just using a little bit less of the oestrogen over longer periods of time.

Women who use HRT oestrogen must also use complementary progestagen hormone so as to protect their womb-lining. However, women who use only the local vaginal oestrogen products do not need additional progestagen. In other words, if you have a womb and use oestrogen that gets into the blood, you also need progestagen. Whereas local vaginal oestrogen does not get into the blood in significant amounts, therefore no progestagen is needed.

The secret to safely using local vaginal oestrogen with minimal absorption into the blood is to use it regularly. If you are experiencing uncomfortable or distressing genito-urinary symptoms and you need vaginal oestrogen to tackle them, you should use as much as you require for as long as you need it. Do not start and stop! You should use a low dose every week for as long as you like to keep the vaginal walls thick and healthy, and this will help to guarantee that as little oestrogen as possible enters the bloodstream.

If you require some form of vagina therapy when you're younger, say in your forties or fifties, the key to ongoing vagina health is to keep using the treatment long-term. For most of the other menopausal symptoms (flushes, sweats, mood, et cetera) you will eventually pass through the transitional phase of the menopause and no longer require hormonal supplements to control symptoms, but this is not true of the vagina. If you don't maintain vagina treatments, things will not balance out and will likely get worse. So, the key to successful use of vagina therapies is to persevere. You don't need to use loads, but you do need to use something, and I'd bet you'll need to for the rest of your senior life. Like I said, some treatments are forever – and that's not a bad thing, you'll be so grateful to have them.

Some high-tech vaginal therapies

This sounds very Obi-Wan Kenobi, but in addition to local hormones there are a variety of types of mechanical treatments emerging that might also help you to cope with some of the problems of a menopausal vagina. For example, a special chair has recently been developed to address continence problems in men and women. The High Intensity Focused Electromagnetic Energy (HIFEM) is used to stimulate and strengthen the pelvic floor muscles. They call it the Emsella chair.

Laser therapy is also of use in treating the vagina and other pelvic structures. Some early work with CO_2 lasers on vaginal wall health showed that while they helped they could cause trauma to the vaginal wall because CO_2 gets hot and can burn you. But all lasers are not the same, and the newer cold lasers (Erbium or ER lasers) don't have that problem. There are a few clinics in Ireland that offer cold laser therapy and it can be very helpful. My friend and vagina guru Dr Rita Galimberti tells me that using vaginal oestrogen after ER laser is usually enough to keep you well without additional laser therapy. She runs a beautiful clinic in west Dublin and there is lots of helpful information on the clinic website (www.femalase.com). Happy zapping!

KEY TAKEAWAYS

- The genito-urinary system is affected by age, among other things, and the effects tends to worsen over time. This means that when you first recognize symptoms, that's the sign to get them checked out. Don't take a 'wait-and-see' attitude.
- If oestrogen depletion is affecting your vagina, you can use local vaginal oestrogen to target those problems directly. It doesn't go through your bloodstream, so it's a safe and effective treatment for most women. But at present, it's not recommended for people who are on aromatase inhibitors (AIs).

6. Early onset menopause arising from hormone issues

Most women will experience a 'natural' menopause, occurring because of aging. It evolves gradually: they may start to skip periods or get occasional symptoms and start to wonder, *Could this be menopause?* They may or may not feel the need to get some advice from their GP. However, some women will face early onset menopause – whether triggered by a medical intervention* or simply due to an ovary hormone deficiency.

It upsets me when women tell me that their early menopause has been treated as no big deal, or even a good thing, by health-care professionals. They have heard things like, 'You've had your children, your family is finished, you weren't going to do anything with those ovaries or that womb anyway.' You'd swear you were having a bit of antique furniture removed! This is the wrong approach because it is a diminution of the role that the pelvic sex organs play in a person's life and identity. So, I'm here to tell you that early onset menopause is a tough gig to face, no matter how it comes about, but there is help out there, once you know how and where to access it.

This chapter focuses on early menopause arising from hormone issues – broadly known as premature ovarian insufficiency (POI; formerly known as premature ovarian failure). This is a situation where a person under forty years of age does not have an adequate supply of ovarian hormone in their body. It is a serious condition that demands medical attention as it is not natural to be lacking female hormone at a young age. On occasion, we see POI in girls who have either delayed or disrupted puberty.

This is a bigger problem than many people realize – about 1 in 100 women will go through menopause before they hit the age of forty,

---

* Such as chemotherapy or hysterectomy or oophorectomy (removal of ovaries).

and 1 in 1,000 will do so before hitting thirty years of age. I've seen seventeen-year-olds who were plunged into menopause, and your heart would absolutely break for them.

Strangely enough, people with POI sometimes report relatively few menopause symptoms, but the ones they do get will be more severe. POI can potentially have a very serious impact on your future health and, if not treated, may even reduce your total life span. A recent study of more than 11,000 Australians with POI found that those women were almost three times more likely to develop cardio-vascular disease (diseases of the heart and blood vessels) in their sixties, as well as having a higher incidence of other chronic conditions, such as osteoporosis.

I am not telling you this to freak you out, but I want to impress upon you that even if you don't feel 'too bad', if you have POI, you need hormone supplements. If you carry on without replacing those hormones, it can increase the risk of some potentially life-limiting conditions. Taking the hormones when you're young will not only make you feel better, it will protect you when you are older. Your senior self will thank you!

What causes premature ovarian insufficiency (POI)

Well, there are many different situations that can give rise to POI. Unfortunately, the majority of people (70 per cent) will never have a reason why this is happening to them, which is extremely frustrat-ing and can create even more upset and anxiety. These are cases of idiopathic POI. 'Idiopathic' means we will never know the reason. *Idio* comes from the Greek, *idios*, which means 'one's own' or 'private', while *pathic* means 'disease', so any disease whose cause is still unknown is referred to as 'idiopathic' by doctors. However, with POI it does seem to run in families, so there is a high probability that we will dis-cover in the future that a gene mutation is at the core of it.

A number of genetic disorders can be linked to POI. These include Down's syndrome, Fragile X syndrome and Turner Syndrome, as well as some other less common genetic disorders.

Auto-immune diseases and infections can also be linked to POI, including conditions such as Hashimoto's disease of the thyroid gland, rheumatoid arthritis, lupus (see Chapter 26), myasthenia gravis, Addison's disease, insulin-dependent diabetes (see Chapter 23), and inflammatory bowel disease (such as Crohn's). Depending on your symptoms, your doctor may do a few tests to rule out these conditions if you present with POI.

Diagnosing POI

Whatever the cause, if you start to experience menopause-type symptoms before you are forty years old, or if your periods have stopped for more than four months and you are under forty – get checked out. If you are deprived of your normal hormones at a young age and it is not corrected, you are at increased risk of reduced fertility, osteoporosis, cardiovascular disease and cognitive impairment, among other things. Therefore, it is essential to seek professional medical help and advice.

When you go to the GP to discuss issues with your menstrual cycle, you should be asked to describe your symptoms, your history and that of your female family members, as well as lifestyle and any medication you are taking. We will ask you to provide some details on your period pattern and, if you are in a heterosexual relationship, we will probably do a pregnancy test because many people skip bleeds for months and then discover they are pregnant. If you do not have a positive pregnancy test, the doctor should examine you to see if there are any other signs that could give clues as to what has happened to your cycle. In this instance, they should also do blood tests to measure your sex hormone levels, as well as other tests, such as an AMH test (see below) if you are trying to get pregnant, to try and either diagnose or exclude POI.* The rules as set down by the European

---

* Here I have to acknowledge that these tests can be hard to access. South Co. Dublin may be the best place in Ireland to access public gynaecological health services via GP and hospital, but other regions are not so well served. If you are having difficulty accessing POI care in your area, speak to your GP about being referred to a dedicated POI service, even if that means a road trip. Most hospital-based POI

Society of Human Reproduction and Embryology (ESHRE) stipu-
late that POI is diagnosed by doing two separate sets of blood tests
at an interval of four to six weeks.

The main hormone of interest is FSH – follicle stimulating hormone. We've already looked at FSH in Chapters 1 and 3, so you're
familiar with it. When the ovary is functioning normally it shuts off
FSH production in the brain, so in most younger women FSH levels
should be low, certainly under 25 IU/L (international units per litre)
and usually more like 5 to15 IU/L – and this is a pretty reliable number.
So, if you're under forty and have elevated FSH levels on two or more
separate occasions about a month apart, chances are you have POI.
How high those levels need to be to diagnose POI depends on what
you read. I have seen values of >25 IU/L in some journals and >45
IU/L in others. Either way, if your levels are high, you need to be
referred to either a hormone specialist (endocrinologist) or a dedicated
gynaecological POI clinic, where possible, to have further evaluation
and hopefully receive advice on treatments and lifestyle options to
maintain well-being and prevent disease and premature death.

Amazingly, about 1 in 4 people with POI will have intermittent
recovery of their ovarian action, so you might ovulate, and if you
are having unprotected sex you might get pregnant. In fact, up to 10
per cent of people with POI conceive spontaneously, so if you are
not seeking a pregnancy and you have suspected or confirmed POI,
you should be using at least barrier contraception like condoms or a
diaphragm.

When the diagnosis of POI is confirmed, we will look for clues in
your family as to why this is happening to you. Then we will check
all the bloods – liver, kidney, thyroid, lipids, sugars, calcium, vitamin
D, et cetera. We might refer you for a DEXA scan to see what your
bone density is like for your age, and maybe a pelvic scan to see what
your womb and ovaries are up to. We will sometimes refer you to
our genetics services to check for inherited disorders that are known
to be connected to POI, especially if you are under thirty, as well as
checking for the many auto-immune conditions that are also linked

clinics run by the HSE do not limit their appointments to patients in their area but
will see people from any of the 26 counties.

to POI. We will also check your history of infections, such as TB, mumps and HIV.

We will sometimes check your ovarian follicle reserve by measuring anti-Müllerian hormone (AMH) levels. AMH is produced in the antral follicles and is somewhat helpful in getting a sense of what that person's egg supply is like. The antral follicle count identifies how many eggs in your ovary are getting ready to be released in ovulation ('antral' comes from *antrum*, which means 'hollow sac'; it refers to the cyst that forms around a maturing egg that has become large enough to see on a scan). Fertile women should have a certain amount of antral follicles at any given time. AMH is not routinely used to diagnose POI, but it may have a role when the diagnosis of POI is inconclusive. It might also be worthwhile doing if you are hoping to get pregnant, as POI can have a major impact on your ability to conceive.

Unsurprisingly, getting a diagnosis of POI can be quite a shock. Depression and low self-esteem are often associated with the diagnosis, and ideally people with POI (like people with any medical condition) should have access to counselling and peer support. In Ireland, it is very hard to access counselling – even when you are paying privately – so online groups are very helpful. One of the best-known and respected POI support organizations is the Daisy Network in the UK: www. daisynetwork.org. There is also an Irish Facebook group hosted by Sallyanne Brady and Claire Peel, called The Irish Menopause, and they often discuss POI-related issues.

Managing POI

I tell my patients with POI that the loss of the natural oestrogen in a young woman is a significant risk factor for quality-of-life reduction, fertility dysfunction and future health issues (particularly cardiovascular disease and osteoporosis, to name only two). However, it is mainly cardiac disease that is the culprit when some women with unmedicated POI are at risk from premature heart disease and death. Accordingly, it is highly recommended to use some form of replacement sex hormones – either HRT or the combined oral contraceptive pill (COCP), patch or ring.

One effect of developing POI is that your personal risk of breast cancer is significantly reduced – a reduction of around 30 per cent when compared to other women in your age range. If you choose to improve your well-being and prevent future important health problems, like early heart attacks, by taking HRT, you lose the benefit of that breast cancer risk reduction. Your personal risk returns to what is normal for women in your age range. This looks like a significant jump but is really just normal for you at your age. All of the menopause societies, in addition to NICE (National Institute for Health and Care Excellence), agree and strongly urge women with unnaturally early oestrogen loss to replace that essential hormone until at least the natural age of menopause. The perceived 'risks' from HRT do not apply unless and until you reach fifty to fifty-five years of age and are still taking HRT.

I really drill into the detail of HRT – what goes into it and the various approaches to taking it – in the dedicated HRT chapters (see Part II), so you will need to read these in tandem with what I'm telling you here. (In fact, it may be useful to read Chapters 9 to 12 now – they're short – and then return to this chapter.) But to keep the flow here, I'll continue with a look at HRT and contraceptive hormones in relation to POI and the needs of people with POI.

Both HRT and a number of contraceptive hormones contain oestrogen and progestagen, so on occasion we give women who need hormonal supplementation the choice of one or the other. In broad terms, HRT might be arguably 'better' for POI, but it really depends on the person and her own health and needs. This is what the British Menopause Society (BMS) has to say on the matter:

> There is limited evidence assessing the optimal regimen, dose or route of administration of hormone replacement in women with POI. HRT and the combined oral contraceptive pill containing ethinylestradiol would both be suitable options for hormone replacement, although HRT may be more beneficial in improving bone health and cardiovascular markers compared to the combined oral contraceptive pill.

Combined hormonal contraceptives (CHC) refers to any of the sixteen-odd pills or the one ring or the one patch available in Ireland that contain both oestrogen and progestagen. 'The pill', as everyone calls it, is a pack of tabs – usually 21 in total, although there are a few brands now that have 28 tabs – that have both progestagen and oestrogen in them. Doctors call these the combined oral contraceptive pills (COCPs) because they contain a combination of oestrogen and progestagen. These are not to be confused with the progestagen-only contraceptive pills (POPs). While POPs are good contraceptives, they contain no oestrogen, so they are not useful for someone who requires oestrogen replacement.

If you have POI and require oestrogen replacement but prefer not to take HRT – and you might in fact benefit from a little contraceptive protection – then you may choose to use CHC to treat POI. Unfortunately, though, the type of hormones usually included in CHC are far stronger and more chemically potent than HRT oestrogen, so not everyone is allowed to use CHC. If, for example, you are quite overweight, are a smoker, or have one of about fifteen different diseases that might make it too risky to be on CHC, then you will only be offered HRT. In that case, you'll have to sort out contraception some other way, like a coil or an implant or even just condoms/ diaphragm – it's your choice.

HRT hormones, especially when the oestrogen goes into the skin, via patch, gel or spray, and is not taken orally, are typically more like the 'natural' oestrogen molecule that the ovaries make. So, if you want as close to natural hormone replacement as possible, HRT is the way to go. Although, once again, it offers no contraceptive protection.

Some people with POI choose to mix it up. They might use the CHC when they are younger and keen not to get pregnant, but then in their thirties they might switch to HRT, especially if they are considering a baby or perhaps exploring fertility support. Whatever you ultimately use to replace your oestrogen, remember that the risks to benefit ratios are not the same for you as they are for other people who make lots of their own oestrogen. You are always better to be on oestrogen than not – certainly until you are fifty-one years old – at which point you may well choose to keep going with HRT. At that point, the pros and cons of HRT are the same for you as they would be for any other menopausal person.

Pros and cons of HRT versus CHC
for a person with POI

HRT	CHC
'Safer' and more 'natural'	Artificially strong hormones – not suitable for all
Almost never causes dangerous side effects when used via patches or spray or gel	Can be linked to blood clots, albeit rarely
Can be pricey for the good stuff	Usually very affordable
Younger women may feel stigmatized being on HRT	Loads of young women are on CHC
Can be tailored to improve sex drive	Not known for improving sex drive, and may impair it
No contraception protection from HRT – and this is important to discuss and be aware of as about 10 to 15 per cent of people with POI can conceive spontaneously	Contraception
May not control bleeds very well	Usually keeps vaginal bleeding light
Won't interfere with getting pregnant	Meant to prevent pregnancy

Sex and POI

Some, but not all, people with confirmed POI have issues surrounding sex. If you feel that you are 'not like other women', this may create some negative self-imagery that is hard to overcome. You might be concerned about the possibility of not easily conceiving and having babies, an anxiety that can affect your sense of yourself as a sexual being. You may have reduced interest in sex and feel less sexual for many reasons, not least of which is the purely physical reason that your underperforming ovaries are not making enough androgen (male hormone) for you to have the usual interest in sex that other people in your age group might enjoy.

The British Menopause Society often gives us updates on a condition associated with typical menopause, known as hypoactive sexual desire disorder/dysfunction (HSDD), which can be linked to the common female sexual arousal disorder (FSAD), whereby a woman notices that her normal interest in sex or her normal arousal and orgasmic enjoyment appear to have switched off. This is more likely to happen when menopause occurs at a young age, therefore POI sufferers are particularly vulnerable to HSDD.

One option for menopausal people – regardless of age – is to add some testosterone to their hormone cocktail. Why testosterone? The male hormones, or androgens, are produced in abundance in the ovary of younger females and are essential for healthy sex drive. Five androgens are found in women, but only one – testosterone – has a direct impact on the body.

The ovaries are the main source of female testosterone. For those with POI who are on HRT oestrogen and progesterone, at the clinic we would offer to add in some form of testosterone to get them back to normal levels for women of their age. Unfortunately, the only form of approved testosterone therapy for females in Ireland has to be imported from Australia, which can really bump up the cost. As a result, GPs and menopause specialists frequently offer the type of testosterone that is normally used in males, but at a much, much lower dosage, thus giving you the testosterone you need at a lower cost. We are warned to be vigilant with testosterone, though, and guidelines require testosterone users to get their blood levels monitored every six to twelve months while they are taking it. (I go into this in detail in Chapter 12.)

What about a little vaginal oestrogen?

Probably! Even though you may be on lashings of oestrogen and progestagen, and even testosterone, your poor vagina and vulva and general pelvic zone may still be crying out for some local oestrogen. As I already described in Chapters 4 and 5, all menopausal women are prone to vulval and vaginal problems. This is particularly the case for those who go into it young. Local oestrogen replacement is not like standard HRT as it only impacts the tissues nearby, in the vicinity of your vagina, and it leaves your womb-lining alone. It is miraculous stuff. Vaginal oestrogen can be used by anyone who needs it, for as long as they need it. If that is forever, that is fine.

Will you need fertility support?

You might. In fact, one of the commonest ways we identify POI in Ireland is when a woman comes in to avail of the fertility services and over the course of testing and treatment the doctors realize she has POI. There are many levels of fertility intervention that are available for people who want to conceive, so there is no way to know for sure what help you may or may not need until you are in the fertility clinic. The time to discuss this, though, is when you are young – maybe long before you are actively trying to get pregnant – so that we can give you more options. So, if you skip months without a period and you are not on a contraceptive that is designed to cause that, see your doctor, get checked out and get some blood tests done, including the ones for POI.

Options we can offer include using HRT cyclically to induce monthly bleeding and hopefully prepare the womb-lining for conception if you do indeed ovulate. Assisted reproduction techniques using the woman's own eggs or donated eggs are available in some private fertility clinics in Ireland. They can freeze and store your own eggs, or your and your partner's embryos, or even ovarian tissue, but success rates will depend on many, many different factors. If you are being treated for a condition that might result in iatrogenic POI – that's POI brought on by medical treatment (see the next chapter) – the time to consider and discuss these options is *before* you start your treatments, assuming you have the luxury of time to do this. There may be limited options for you if you undergo a therapy that damages your eggs or womb and you have not received some advice beforehand. If no one mentions this to you, *you* need to start that conversation.

KEY TAKEAWAYS

- ☒ POI is serious and needs to be corrected with hormonal supplementation, wherever possible.
- ☒ If you have high FSH and you are under forty, you should be referred to a dedicated POI service or a hospital clinic that specializes in POI.
- ☒ The earlier you get assessed, the better, so as to get on treatment that will help to maintain your health and optimize your fertility options.
- ☒ Reach out to local POI support groups because there are many other people out there going through the same stuff as you – it is good to talk!

7. Early onset menopause arising from medical treatment

There are many different situations where you can lose ovary hormones quite quickly and end up with POI – overnight in some cases – and these are usually after medical interventions. Menopause as a result of medical treatments is called *iatrogenic* menopause. It comes from the Greek word *iatros*, meaning 'doctor', so it's 'doctor-caused' menopause. This can come about through surgery, radiation or a medication that knocks out your normally functional ovaries. The combination of chemotherapy and radiotherapy for cancers such as Hodgkin lymphoma is associated with the highest incidence of iatrogenic POI.

Giving a woman a treatment that causes early menopause is something we doctors should never do lightly, and then only with all the right supports in place. Ideally, all women who may be facing an iatrogenic menopause, for whatever reason, should have a long consultation and some counselling about what the treatment will do to them and what choices they have about managing those symptoms.

Surgical procedures that bring on menopause

Some women will be advised to have one or both of their ovaries removed in a procedure known as an oophorectomy. This may be because of gynaecological cancers (especially cervical and ovarian), severe endometriosis, premenstrual dysphoric disorder (PMDD) and diseases of the ovaries, such as severe ovarian cysts, ovarian cancer, twisted ovary (torsion) and ovarian abscess. That's not an exhaustive list, but those conditions are common causes. Some blood disorders may also be managed by removing the ovaries. Even when you are left with one ovary, you might still develop earlier menopause symptoms because of the impact of the surgery on blood flow in the pelvis. (See Chapter 18 for detailed material about breast cancer and menopause.)

Alternatively, you may be at risk of certain diseases and the operation is recommended to try to avoid that. For example, women who are known to carry the breast cancer or BRCA gene mutation (or other cancer genes) or women who appear to have cancer syndromes, such as Lynch syndrome (an inherited disease associated with colorectal cancer as well as cancers of the womb, ovaries, stomach, liver, kidney, brain and skin), may be advised to have their ovaries (and sometimes breasts or womb) removed because they have a higher than usual risk of cancers in these parts of the body. This kind of operation, aimed at reducing their risk, is called *prophylactic* or risk-reducing surgery.

Whatever your personal situation, it is imperative that you and your surgeon discuss the after-effects of removing the ovaries *before* you have the operation. 'Just talk to your GP if you feel unwell after the op' is, in my opinion, BS and simply not good enough any more – not that it ever was. Typically, the menopause symptoms that happen following ovary removal surgery are immediate and severe. You might wake up from the anaesthetic with significant symptoms that require immediate care. So, some form of hormone or non-hormone treatment plan needs to be in place before they operate on you.

This discussion and preplanning are even more imperative when considering removing the ovaries in women under the age of forty, as this is an induced premature menopause, which, as you saw in the previous chapter, can lead to all kinds of serious health issues if not carefully managed.

Menopause brought on by drug therapies

Some women are advised to undergo treatments for cancers (and other serious disorders) that can bring on many side effects, which are often related to ovarian tissue destruction or oestrogen hormone impairment. When menopause symptoms are brought on by these medications, we call it chemical menopause.

Cancer chemotherapy

These regimens are used to shrink and destroy cancer cells in the blood and tissues. As cancer cells tend to grow and reproduce very quickly – compared to normal cells – cancer specialists (oncologists) often recommend a course of chemotherapy because it kills fast-growing cells, hopefully without killing too many normal, healthy cells. Unfortunately, most cancer chemotherapy drugs can harm the ovaries by damaging the ovarian tissue and blood vessels.

Cancer adjuvant therapy

This is often recommended in women who have been diagnosed with breast cancer, usually after they have had surgery and/or a chemo-therapy regime. The word *adjuvant* means 'helping' or 'contributing'. The two main types of breast cancer adjuvant therapy are aromatase inhibitors and Tamoxifen. These can both induce menopausal symptoms but they work in different ways.

AROMATASE INHIBITORS

AI therapy is used in the treatment of oestrogen receptor positive breast cancer. (All cells have receptors on them – that is how they talk to each other.) They are usually prescribed for women who are older and no longer menstruating, but there are many other situations in which AI therapy is recommended.

AIs work by blocking a chemical process called aromatization. Why does that help reduce breast cancer spread and recurrence? Well, in older women whose natural ovarian hormone production is very low, most of the oestrogen in their bloodstream comes from other places in their body, like their breasts, brain, liver and skin. In those tissues there will be low levels of testosterone floating around, which get changed to oestrogens through a chemical process known as aromatization. The enzyme aromatase is required to make that chemical reaction happen. AIs block aromatase activity, which means less testosterone being converted into estrone and estradiol, thereby reducing the amount of oestrogen in the blood, which in turn means there is less oestrogen to feed the tumour cells in oestrogen receptor positive cancers.

Unfortunately, though, AIs can have unwanted side effects, particularly: persistent joint and muscle pain, flushes, sweats, sleep problems, et cetera. These would go away if you took oestrogen through HRT, but that would make no sense as the whole point of the AI is to reduce the amount of oestrogen in the blood. This is why we usually look to non-HRT strategies to help women with AI side effects.

TAMOXIFEN

This belongs to a class of hormones known as a SERM — selective oestrogen receptor modulator. SERMs have been around for years and come in many different types, but they all have the ability to block the oestrogen receptors on some tissues, and also (amazingly) to stimulate oestrogen receptors on other tissues. That's why they have 'selective' in their title. They are often used in women with breast cancer, particularly if they are still menstruating. The blocking effect of the Tamoxifen on the oestrogen receptor positive breast cancer cells prevents cancer growth and recurrence.

Unfortunately, most SERMs, including Tamoxifen, block oestrogen receptors on tissues such as the skin, bladder, vagina and brain. They can cause menopausal symptoms, such as joint pain, hot flushes, fatigue, mood swings and depression, dry skin, loss of libido, et cetera. Tamoxifen does not reduce the amount of oestrogen floating around the bloodstream like AIs do — instead, it blocks the effects of oestrogen on many cell receptors. This seems to cause worse menopause symptoms for most users than AI medications do.

Again, we are not meant to offer HRT to women on Tamoxifen because it is counterproductive to the goal of shutting down the oestrogen receptors on the breast cancer cells — but there are many other things we can try in its place. For example, women on Tamoxifen are often offered cognitive behavioural therapy (CBT), SSRIs and SNRIs (anti-depressants), oxybutynin or gabapentin for their menopause symptoms, instead of systemic HRT (see the next chapter for non-medical alternatives to HRT). In addition, Tamoxifen users can also use vaginal HRT.

GnRH analogue injections

These induce a chemical menopause for the three months for which each injection lasts. GnRH injections cause ovarian 'shut-down' by activating the luteinizing hormone (LH) receptors in the brain that signal the ovaries to stop making oestrogen. They are mainly used short-term to block ovarian activity, which benefits conditions like PMDD, heavy menstrual bleeding and bleeding fibroids. They are also used in IVF preparation and for ovarian suppression in trans-gender men. But they bring on quite dramatic menopausal symptoms in most cases, and some form of add-back hormone therapy will usually be offered alongside.

When radiotherapy targets the pelvis or lower abdomen

This can arise for women who have to undergo radiotherapy for cancers. In radiotherapy, ionizing radiation is delivered using high-energy beams from sources such as X-rays, electron beams, proton beams and gamma rays, all of which destroy fast-growing cells near the area where the radiation is directed. As cancer cells tend to grow very fast, those cells are destroyed more quickly than the surrounding healthy tissues. Nonetheless, some normal cells in the area can also be damaged by radiotherapy and this can cause a multitude of side effects. When radiation therapy is directed into the pelvis or lower abdomen, it is more likely to damage the ovaries and may well affect their function. And even when radiation is targeted outside the pelvis, the ovaries sometimes still suffer as the radiation can be absorbed by distant tissues.

How much damage will it cause? That is hard to predict, because it will depend on things like the amount and type of radiation given. In some cases, the reproductive organs can be 'temporarily relocated' outside the pelvis so as to avoid the worst of the radiotherapy. After the radiation treatment ends, the surgeons can then replace your womb and ovaries back into your pelvis and hopefully preserve the function and your fertility.

I have a great story about my buddy, an oncology surgeon, who treated a young woman with bowel cancer. She needed pelvic radiation but wanted to preserve her fertility. He performed a surgery and relocated her womb next to her liver and brought her cervical opening out through her belly button so she could keep having periods. She managed them by sticking a sanitary pad over the belly button. And you might be thinking: *Wait, wouldn't the body reject that alien relocation?* But no, it's still your own tissue, so the body doesn't care (the body is cool like that!). When the bowel surgery was treated and in remission, he put it all back where it belonged. Just amazing.

Early menopause is tough – hang in there

All in all, it can be a rough road when you receive a diagnosis of POI, or you're told a medical treatment is going to plunge you into early menopause, and you need to grab all the help you can get. You'll manage it so much better if you are well informed and well supported. Not everyone has the wherewithal to be in charge of their own care but doing some reading and asking informed questions of your doctors and nurses is key to getting as good an outcome as you can. I hope these two chapters have given you a solid basis for understanding POI and framing your questions and concerns for your health-care provider. I've lived through a natural menopause myself, and even that was pretty rough, no lying, but I made it over the line and out the other side, so I know it can be done.

KEY TAKEAWAYS

☒ If you are facing surgery or medical treatment that is likely to cause menopause, you must discuss this with your medical team well in advance. It's important that a treatment plan is in place to help you manage your symptoms from the outset.

☒ If your specialist does not mention it, ask for information!

☒ If the treatment you will undergo includes being prescribed AIs or Tamoxifen, that creates a particular set of circumstances that must be managed carefully. Again, you need to have a full and frank discussion with your medical team to figure out your best options for managing your menopause symptoms safely.

☒ It is essential to ask for information on side effects, including menopause symptoms, that could occur before, during and after your cancer treatment. (See www.arccancersupport.ie for information and advice.)

PART II
Managing the symptoms of perimenopause and menopause

8. Non-HRT treatment options for menopause symptoms

As you'll have gathered, I am a fan of HRT. Modern HRT provides an excellent, safe and reliable way to tackle the symptoms of peri-menopause and menopause. It is my preferred choice to deal with my own symptoms. However, most women do not take HRT, either because they don't have bad symptoms or they are happy to manage their symptoms in other ways, and that is great – HRT is not supposed to be thrown around like Smarties! You should not feel *less than* or worried if you don't need it, or if you have no choice and can't take it. You might also have a deep-seated resistance to messing around with what you see as Mother Nature's plan for you, and I respect that – nobody should feel railroaded into using something that doesn't feel right to them. In fact, I tease out the various aspects of HRT in this book *precisely because* I recognize that women have all kinds of legitimate practical and indeed philosophical concerns about it, so the more you know the better. While I am unapologetic and passionate about encouraging women not to suffer needlessly (and I have seen too much of this in my decades in practice), I am not trying to persuade women to go on HRT if they don't want to. My aim is not to persuade but to make sure you have the fullest possible information when arriving at your decision. It's about empowerment!

Before moving on to talk about HRT in detail, I want to look at other options for managing symptoms and also to examine some of the claims made for 'natural' remedies.* It is important that, whatever you choose, you're getting your symptoms dealt with, you are safe, and

---

* There are also prescription meds that can be given instead of HRT for people who can't use it. The British Menopause Society (BMS) provides information and guidelines on non-hormonal treatments. Practitioners may wish to refer to the online resources listed at the back of the book.

you're getting your money's worth. This chapter explores the options that some people try and looks at where we are now (approaching the mid-2020s) vis-à-vis the science of risk versus benefit of those alternatives to HRT.

The non-prescription options for managing symptoms of perimenopause are lumped together in a group called 'complementary therapies'. We can break that down into three types:

- **Foods/dietary products**: this includes diet supplements and vitamins, herbs, probiotics, et cetera
- **Physical therapies and treatments**: such as acupuncture/ acupressure, yoga, massage, spinal manipulation and laser vaginal therapies
- **Psychological therapies**: such as cognitive behavioural therapy (CBT), mindfulness and other meditations, relaxation therapies, hypnotherapy, among others.

Food and the other stuff you put in your body

Prepare to roll your eyes because what follows here is a familiar recital of the principles of healthy eating. But it is the case that optimizing general health and nutrition may help lessen some of the impact of the menopause. I mean, it's got to be worth at least considering ditching the chocolate biscuits if it helps!

The changes the body is going through during perimenopause and menopause can result in weight gain for some people. This is due to the slowing down of your metabolism as you age and the fact that our bodies shift from gluteo-femoral (buttocks and thighs) to central adipose deposition – in other words, belly fat. Weight gain can have other side effects, including tiredness and low mood. That can create a vicious circle: you're tired, you're feeling low, what's going to help?

Chocolate! Ice cream! Wine!

We all know how that goes. Eating well isn't hard, in theory, but it can be very hard when you're feeling crap to begin with and down on yourself – then, it's an uphill battle. I think it helps to break it down into some daily habits that you can manage pretty easily.

Let's recap on what works for your body in terms of an easy enough daily healthy diet.

- *Eating oily fish, low sugar fruits and vegetables, whole grains, soya, legumes*, et cetera, all of which reduce bad cholesterol. This is a time of life when you really need to get bad cholesterol under control, which should be the guideline for your eating.
- *Keeping your blood sugar under control.* A handy way to be aware of sugar content is to use the glycaemic index (GI), which tells us how fast certain foods raise your glucose (blood sugar) level. If you stick to low GI foods, that's beneficial for your body and will help with weight control as well. (You could check out the Diabetes Ireland website at www.diabetes.ie for an introduction to the GI.)
- *Avoiding excess red meat and simple sugars* can help in controlling your weight and in reducing hot flushes.
- *Taking vitamin D daily*, at least 400mIU/day, will improve your bone health, which is always a concern as oestrogen drops and hormones fluctuate. Generally, I prefer people to eat their vitamins but I think for Irish people, where everyone needs more vitamin D, supplements are particularly advisable in wintertime (since it's created by exposing the skin to sunlight, and we don't get enough sun year round).
- *Making sure to get calcium every day*. Calcium is best taken in via food in a calcium-rich diet. No one needs a calcium supplement unless they are on bone medications or have a calcium restricted diet – like lactose intolerant people, for example – but for anyone with a low calcium diet, taking calcium daily, around 700–1,200mg/day, may be useful. Sources of calcium in food include all forms of dairy, calcium-fortified drinks, canned fish – especially salmon with the bones left in (yuk!) – spinach, beans, tofu and figs.
- *Reducing or even eliminating booze.* Heavy alcohol consumption is linked to increased rates of breast cancer, low bone density, falls and fractures, and more. The official recommendation, according

to the HSE, is 11 units per week for women and 14 for men. This is not your weekly target – this is the maximum amount, and you should be aiming to be well under it. Really, the recommendation is zero alcohol because alcohol adds nothing beneficial to our bodies – it's got no reason to be there at all. It's interesting to note that while in Ireland it's recommended that women keep alcohol intake under 11 standard drinks a week, in the USA the Centers for Disease Control and Prevention (CDC) recommends women to stay under 7 units per week. It's helpful to check out the online Drinkaware calculator at https://drinkaware.ie/drinks-calculator/.

• *Stopping smoking.* Smoking affects every inch of your body, inside and out. Hard as it is for smokers to hear, you really have to cut down and ideally stop completely – and that includes vaping. It's not easy to do, but it really is worth it. If you give up smoking, it:

~ improves sleep, hair, skin and teeth quality;
~ improves your exercise capacity, endurance and enjoyment;
~ improves fertility for both men and women;
~ increases your potential life span by 10–15 years;
~ reduces your risk of heart disease, emphysema, lung cancer, throat cancer, mouth cancer, bladder cancer, breast cancer, thrombosis, stomach ulcers, and more;
~ reduces your risk of death from heart disease by 50 per cent within six months.

Just read that back over: *increases your life span by 10–15 years* – that's a whole lot of life you'd get to live and hopefully enjoy. And *reduces risk of death from heart disease by 50 per cent after just six months* – knowing, as we do, how our risk of heart disease jumps up after menopause, that's a powerful statistic. If you smoke, you're risking a lesser life and a potentially longer and harder road to death, via disease of one kind or another. You owe it to yourself to ditch the cigarettes. Smoking cessation is hard, though – ask your doctor or pharmacist for help. See the HSE's dedicated website at www.quit.ie.

A note on veganism/vegetarianism and menopause

A person with a balanced vegetarian or vegan diet approaching their mid-life should be no more prone to oestrogen imbalance and deficiency symptoms or future medical conditions, such as heart disease, bone loss and cognitive decline, than someone who has an omnivorous diet. There may in fact be protection there: some small-sized surveys have reported that menopause symptoms are less troublesome in some women who have a plant-based diet.

If, however, you are nutritionally lacking in certain vitamins, minerals and proteins, you may be more exposed to other medical problems, such as osteoporosis (thinning bones) and sarcopaenia (reduced muscle mass). So, make sure you are taking in adequate dietary calcium and protein, and consider a daily vitamin D supplement.*

A note on cholesterol and menopause

Cholesterol is an essential molecule that is found in every cell in the body. We use cholesterol to make hormones like oestrogen, progesterone and vitamin D. We also use it to make bile acids in the liver that will absorb fats during digestion. So, we need some cholesterol, but not too much – or at least not too much of the less helpful types of cholesterol, i.e. the 'bad' cholesterol. Cholesterol is an umbrella term – your total cholesterol consists of:

- **LDL cholesterol (or low-density lipoprotein)**: this is the bad cholesterol. This is the crap that plays a role in plaque build-up in your arteries. It sticks to the lining of your arteries, like a scum ring on the bath, and once there it causes the lining of the artery to become 'inflamed'. The body sends inflammation-fighting cells to the area to contain the threat, and this results in the formation of permanent plaques, or blockages, in the artery.

---

* While I'm on the topic of veganism – and going off the theme of non-HRT approaches to dealing with menopause symptoms – vegans regularly ask me about whether or not they can use HRT. There are issues around this: for example, all oestrogen only and oestrogen + progestagen tablets contain lactose. If you are vegan and looking into the HRT option, you can ask your HRT provider for details on this.

- **HDL cholesterol (or high-density lipoprotein)**: we need some of this stuff as we think it keeps the LDL levels low.
- **Triglycerides (TGL)**: these are another type of lipid, or fat, found in the blood. In women, TGL levels seem to be especially linked to increased risk for heart disease when compared with men. Triglycerides are a source of energy, but elevated TGL levels are linked to increased risk of cardiovascular disease. It's possible that, like LDLs, TGLs may contribute to plaque formation. Excess alcohol, too many simple carbohydrates (sugary and starchy foods), saturated fats (found in meat and dairy products) and trans fats (industrial fats created in factories and used in processed foods) are shown to increase TGL.

We know that up until menopause, LDL cholesterol levels are lower and HDL cholesterol levels are higher in women when you compare them to men of the same age. Then, when menopause hits, LDL cholesterol levels start to climb for most women, often going even higher than men of their same age. Plus, our good HDL cholesterol levels start to go down after menopause. Some of this is hormonal, but some of it is genetic – so if you have a gene for crazy bad cholesterol, you're going to need lipid-lowering drugs, aka statins.

Supplements

Herbal remedies seem to promise the sun, moon and stars to menopausal women. You'll be in the supermarket or pharmacy, and you'll be sorely tempted – especially if they promise to reduce or clear symptoms. Or you might have that one friend who looks great and puts it all down to some alternative thing she discovered online and that 'absolutely works'. Some of the better-known ones include black cohosh, ginseng, evening primrose oil, dong quai (sometimes called the 'female ginseng'), gingko biloba, sage, wild yam and St John's wort. It can melt your head trying to navigate between all the options and decide where to spend your hard-earned cash.

I am a conventional doctor, working in a profession where we are bound by lots of codes of practice, but the biggest one is *Primum non nocere – First, do no harm.*★ I may not make you better, but I must strive to minimize risk and avoid harming you – that is the goal. I need to be confident that something will not just help you long-term but will also be safe for you all the time you are taking it. When it comes to non-HRT menopausal products, the British Menopause Society (BMS) and the National Institute for Health and Care Excellence (NICE) offer some guidance on this topic, and they say there is mixed evidence on the effectiveness of some products – and no evidence at all on others. Most of the herbal remedies and supplements I've mentioned already are probably safe (but see some cautions further down) but have not yet been proven effective.

Phytoestrogens are naturally occurring plant compounds that are similar to estradiol (the principal form of oestrogen released by the ovary that acts on oestrogen receptors in the body) and can have oestrogenic and/or anti-oestrogenic effects on the body. They can be found in beans and peas, chickpeas, lentils, wholegrain cereals, wheatgerm, et cetera. Lignans, a sub-group of phytoestrogens, are found in bran, flax and legumes (for example, peas, beans, lentils). And you can buy them in supplement form in health food shops. *Red clover extract* is a well-known example.

While there may be some benefit to be gained by trying the food sources, the more concentrated source of phytoestrogen will be supplements. However, the few studies available on phytoestrogen supplementation do not really show much by way of benefit over the placebo effect. The BMS says:

> Most studies evaluating effectiveness of phytoestrogens are of poor quality and were not shown to reduce hot flush frequency. Data on phytoestrogen safety and survival benefits in breast cancer patients are inconsistent and as they are known to have oestrogenic activities, isoflavones including Red Clover are not recommended for breast cancer survivors.

Isoflavones are chemical compounds that are usually derived from plants. As well as red clover, they are found in legumes such as

---

★ There is no evidence that Hippocrates ever uttered these apocryphal words. And Irish doctors do not take such an oath. But the basic idea is sound.

soybeans, chickpeas and tofu. They can both stimulate and block oestrogen receptors in the body, and are also recommended for the relief
of sweats and flushes. In my own practice, because there have been
no large-scale studies conducted to look at phytoestrogens when it
comes to their safety or their effectiveness, I do not routinely recommend them. My advice is that anyone who has been told to avoid
HRT oestrogen should probably not be using too much of this stuff
either, just in case.

Black cohosh is sometimes recommended for relief of sweats and
flushes. It too has oestrogen-like effects in the body, so it stands to
reason that it might ease flushes and sweats. But how much is a safe
dose? And could it have an impact on breast cancer recurrence? We just
don't know. The BMS say that while some studies show that black
cohosh can help relieve vasomotor flushes and sweats, it is also associated with side effects, such as constipation, stomach cramps, heart
rhythm disorders and weight gain. Most importantly, it interferes with
the breast cancer drug Tamoxifen and so **must not be used by people
using that medicine**.

That is also the case for *St John's wort*. It has been shown to be effective for both menopausal flushing and low mood. It may impair the
activity of other medications as it is a liver enzyme-inducing drug.
Therefore, people on certain cancer drugs, hormonal contraception
or HRT need to avoid it. And, again, **women who are being treated
for breast cancer with Tamoxifen must not take St John's wort**.

Ginseng is often recommended for menopause symptoms, but the
BMS states that ginseng and Chinese herbal medicines (for example,
dong quai, ginkgo biloba) have not been shown to improve hot flushes,
anxiety or low mood.

The mineral *magnesium* is being studied at the moment, although
not for flushes, only for its effect on sleeping patterns and restless leg
syndrome. So, there are no actual recommendations yet. I would err
on the side of caution and hold off taking it until recommendations
are compiled, based on clinical studies.

Wild yam, sage, maca, pollen extract, vitamin E, evening primrose oil . . .
there is as yet no evidence to show that any of these help with menopausal symptoms. (Evening primrose oil helps with breast pain in some
circumstances – we use it for people with PMS, for example.) Most

importantly, if you look at the breast cancer info pages, they often warn women on breast cancer meds to avoid these 'natural remedies' as there can be a conflict with their breast cancer drugs. So, I would urge women who are post-breast cancer to be very aware of this and cautious about what they take.

There are many vitamin supplements that claim to help relieve menopause symptoms – they often have the word 'meno' right in the brand name. We do know that many people might be deficient in certain minerals and vitamins and that this can affect their general health. However, in terms of menopause symptoms, vitamins have never been shown to control symptoms or prevent oestrogen depletion diseases the way HRT can.

That said, as I mentioned already, anyone living through a winter in Ireland could probably do with some supplemental *vitamin D*. And if you have dietary issues or choose to avoid certain categories of foods (say, if you're vegan), you might need some B-complex vitamins. When it comes to using vitamins, I'd suggest you buy a cheap multivitamin and use that as a general health supplement, but I wouldn't recommend a vitamin supplement as your primary method of controlling menopause symptoms.

Please do not assume that just because something is available over the counter, in a pharmacy or in a health food shop, it is safer or more 'natural' than standard HRT – it isn't. Pharmaceutical companies cannot advertise in Ireland, so you will never hear a radio or TV ad for HRT (like they have in the USA), but you will hear ads for some non-HRT menopause products because they are not subject to the same rules. Wild mushrooms, rhubarb leaves, belladonna (deadly nightshade) and foxgloves grow naturally all over Ireland, but I would not consider eating them because I know they might harm me – just because something is natural doesn't mean it's safe!

Physical therapies and treatments

Prepare to roll your eyes once more as I again state the obvious! *Exercise* is the most straightforward and immediate physical therapy available. Alongside your healthy eating habits, it's wise to get in exercise every week – or every day, if you can, as you get older. Carving out the time can be challenging, of course, at a busy time in your life, but even a brisk walk is worthwhile (that's if you are not impaired in any way – it might, for example, trigger the fibromyalgia ladies). The World Health Organization recommends 75 minutes of vigorous or 150 minutes of moderate aerobic exercise *per week* (that's about 11 to 21 minutes a day of exercise that gets your heart rate up slightly). The benefits of exercise are proven and very convincing:

- decreases premature death, heart disease, diabetes, high blood pressure, colon cancer, obesity and more
- has a beneficial effect on bone and muscle, and can reduce the risk of falling by improving strength, flexibility and balance
- improves most psychological symptoms
- reduces bad cholesterol and raises good cholesterol.

If you can't walk or swim or cycle, ask your GP or physiotherapist for help. There may be ways to allow you to be 'active' when conventional exercise is denied to you.

Apart from exercise, again you'll come across a number of over-the-counter products and gadgets in the pharmacy that may or may not help you manage your menopause. Although, in general, I do not recommend them (because their efficacy hasn't been clinically proven), some of what's out there is plain old common sense and very helpful. For example, using a fan to cool you off during a hot flush is practical and it works. I still sleep with a fan on every night, which I started doing almost twenty years ago when my symptoms started. By this stage, I just like the white noise. But keeping your environment on the cooler side, especially when you are in bed, is smart. You can always throw another blanket on the bed, but you can only peel off so much. Windows open and fans on, I say! Likewise, a little desk fan at work makes total sense.

Some women find their own ingenious solutions – a woman I saw in the clinic recently was telling me that she lies down on her kitchen floor tiles before going to bed, to get her skin as cold as possible so that she can fall asleep. Whatever works for you, go for it! Layered clothing is also a no-brainer.

I have seen special waterproof make-up that is hot flush/ sweat-proof – genius.

As for an €80 magnet that sticks to your underpants to balance your hormone energies? There is absolutely no evidence to support this. On the other hand, it is unlikely to do much harm, so it's not a bad thing per se, and if you want to try it out, that's fine. But be aware that a magnet in your pants can have unwanted consequences – like drawing metal objects across a table to your nether regions during a work meeting (true story!). I also had a friend who had to fish her magnet out of a toilet bowl when she dropped it in there after a little too much vino.

The thing to remember is that you might get short-term relief from symptoms when you start using something – this is the placebo effect. The brain is a powerful thing and if you believe something will help, it just might. (I was at a talk where the speaker described how meeting a doctor or nurse who listens and fills you with hope helps to alleviate short-term symptoms – the brain is so incredible!) Your own hope and positivity can make you feel better. Keep monitoring the effects and be honest with yourself as to whether something is working or not – or was working and isn't any longer. You are trying to manage what could be a difficult set of symptoms, so you have to level with yourself and admit if something was a bad buy. It's trial and error – don't worry about admitting the error and moving on. Because the truth is that, sadly, all the placebo effect in the world – or all the magnets – will not protect your bones and brain and heart if you are oestrogen-deprived. You need HRT for that.

In Chapter 5 I mentioned *vaginal lasers for GSM*. There is emerging research that laser therapy, particularly cold laser treatments, could help with GSM symptoms. At present the volume of clinical evidence for their use is on the low side so it's a wait-and-see situation to see how effective laser therapy is.

A time for self-care – the benefits of psychological therapies

Cognitive behavioural therapy (CBT), mindfulness and other forms of meditation, relaxation therapies, hypnotherapy, all of these are a good idea. When you enter the menopause spectrum, it's a good time for self-care, and minding your mental health and stress levels is part of that. This is the 'silver lining' aspect of reaching the later years in your life – you might have been ignoring yourself for years as you forged a career, or created a home, or took care of children or elderly relatives, or dealt with ill health – or all of the above, whatever life has thrown at you. Indeed, you may still be juggling many of these responsibilities.

Even if life remains full-on, the changes in your body will cause a natural change in outlook and priorities. And you can start to see this change of life as your chance to reframe things – slow down a bit, take stock, look at the bigger picture of your life, prepare yourself for aging as best you can. Psychological therapies come under that umbrella and can be helpful in managing this new phase.

Cognitive Behavioural Therapy (CBT)

Many studies have looked at CBT and its impact on flushes and have shown excellent results. This is particularly the case in cancer clinics, where HRT is generally not an easy option and so they rely quite heavily on CBT, and it can really help.

CBT is a blanket term to describe the many different techniques we can try to make improvements in the way we think and behave and how we feel emotionally and physically by first understanding that it is all interconnected. Our minds are so powerful that we can physically change how we feel in body and mind and spirit by becoming aware of how we respond to our world – what thoughts trigger negative feelings and behaviours – and then how we can retrain our brains to respond in a different way. CBT helps you to look at your life and your ways of responding to the world around you – which can get very stressful at times, especially when menopause is kicking your butt – and to be able to say, *I know I feel like this, but can I turn that around? Can I respond with less anger/fear/defeat and be more accepting of things I cannot change?*

A hot flush is a good example of how CBT can help you to cope. The experience of a hot flush can be very disturbing. Mine usually start from around my knees – I feel a tingling and a heat that rapidly rolls along my thighs and into my pelvis, buzzing and vibrating around my bladder and back passage, and then up along my abdomen and chest into my armpits and neck and right up to the top of my scalp. I become visibly red and the sweating that follows starts as a little sheen, but without my HRT it can build up rapidly to full-blown dripping sweat from my temples, my top lip, between my breasts. Sometimes, my shirt becomes stained with perspiration and, in the beginning, I wasn't a hundred per cent sure that I wasn't having a heart attack! And, of course, this can happen twenty times a day and throughout the night, when it wakes you from sleep and naturally produces a little panic reaction!

Using CBT, at its absolute most basic level, you try to learn to embrace the process, so instead of saying, *Oh cripes, here we go, this is going to be awful*, et cetera, you rewrite the script to say something like, *Oh hello, Miss Flush! I know who you are, I know what you are, and I know I am not going to die from a heart attack. I know that you will roll over me for the next few minutes and I won't fight you, old friend, you do what you need to do. I might just slowly slip this jacket off or grab a drink of cold water and let you pass. You do what you need to do and I will welcome you and enjoy you for what you are.* It's an approach that used to remind me of early labour contractions – they hurt, but I welcomed them. I was delighted to have them because I knew they were not dangerous, that I was not going to die from them, and that this was the start of the birth I had been waiting nine long months to experience.

CBT helps you retrain your response to your menopause symptoms. It allows you to acknowledge it's happening and to greet it with, *Let's ride* – leaning into the experience, as it were.

Of course, this is a gross over-simplification of CBT because a lot of the negative thoughts, feelings and ultimately behaviours we have as humans come from feeling unworthy and judged and embarrassed. Flushes in public can be hard to deal with, no matter your mental outlook, because you feel people are looking at you – and they are. I have had kind strangers ask me if I'm okay during a flush, if they can get me some water, leaving me red as much with embarrassment as with heat!

Now though, having done some CBT training myself, I have retrained my own thoughts and feelings surrounding hot flushes. Thanks to HRT they rarely happen to me any more, but when they do, I always greet the telltale tingling as an old friend, accept it, and if I'm around people I say to them, 'Give me a minute, please, I am having some menopause flushing. It'll just take a minute to ride this out and then we can carry on.' I'm able to say that without shame or embarrassment or fear of judgement because, after all: *Too damn bad about you, world!*

This is what I think psychological therapies, including CBT, can do for you. You learn to say: *This is my reality, and I am doing the best I can, we all struggle, I struggle, but I am no longer going to try to hide it or be ashamed of the struggle. I am going to talk about it and normalize it and embrace it.*

You'll be a happier person if you can do this. Amen.

Non-HRT prescription meds

Finally, there are also prescription meds that can be used instead of HRT. I'm basing the information here on BMS guidelines on non-hormonal treatments. These meds have been used with some effect and may give some symptom relief to people who are advised to avoid HRT.

- *Clonidine* – could reduce hot flushes.
- *SSRIs and SNRIs (anti-depressants)* – could reduce hot flushes, but are **not recommended for those taking Tamoxifen**.
- *Gabapentin and pregabalin* – could reduce hot flushes, and gabapentin is on the list of meds that can relieve restless leg syndrome.
- *Oxybutynin* – could reduce hot flushes.

These are possible alternatives that might suit you – but you'll need to discuss it in detail with your GP

And . . . the future

Your body is full of receptors that act like a complicated signalling system, responding to all kinds of external and internal stimuli, helping it to function (or sometimes, malfunction). Research is being conducted into neurokinin B, a receptor that interacts with the temperature-controlling centre in the brain. In post-menopausal women oestrogen deficiency increases neurokinin B so that the pathway is overstimulated, leading to flushes and sweats. Agents – or 'antagonists' – that act against this receptor could suppress the pathway and thereby reduce flushes and sweats.

Early results are promising but further studies are required, and are under way. The possibility of an effective, safe, non-hormonal option for women who cannot, or prefer not to, take HRT is an exciting prospect for the future. They are starting to recruit patients in Ireland very soon, and women who have been treated for breast cancer can participate. I cannot wait to see if these are as good as they promise – could be a game-changer for us all.

KEY TAKEAWAYS

- Not everybody going through menopause will need or want hormone replacement therapy (HRT).
- Many women have found relief in non-prescription therapies; some but not all of them have been proven to be beneficial and safe.
- It is your choice. But be sure to inform yourself before you make the choice, to make sure that it is the right choice for you.
- If you have health issues (like breast cancer) that could be made worse by using the female hormones in HRT, there are a few medical therapies that can offer relief from some, but not all, of your menopause symptoms – and more are coming soon. Hold tight!

9. An overview of HRT

Of all the methods of managing your menopause symptoms the best known, and perhaps least understood, is HRT. We've all heard of it, but do you have a solid understanding of what it is – make-up, pros and cons – or really just a clutch of anecdotes and a general uneasy sense that it's 'not good' to be on HRT? That was very much the case up until about seven years ago, but it's changing now, I'm glad to say. At the clinic I still meet women who are resistant to the idea of HRT, but when I drill down into their reasons, it really boils down to a niggling worry that 'they say' HRT causes breast cancer. (I explore the origins of these fears at the end of this chapter.)

I can tell you that HRT has moved on by leaps and bounds in the last three decades and now provides a very effective and reliable way of managing menopause symptoms. I depend on my own HRT patch for sanity and quality of life. It's a strong and useful option when symptoms are getting in the way of you enjoying your life.

In this chapter and the next four chapters I'm going to set out exactly what HRT is, the different types available, and the benefits and side effects of each type. This way, you'll be fully informed with up-to-date information that will help you in making decisions about your own menopause and what, if any, treatment path you might choose.

The clue to how HRT works is in the name.* As you discovered in Part I, the symptoms of the menopause are caused by fluctuating and then falling levels of ovarian hormones. When we say HRT, we are talking about products that replace or supplement the sex hormone

---

* I should also note a forthcoming name change: we are now encouraged to rename HRT as MHT – Menopausal Hormone Therapy. The word 'replacement' helps perpetuate the misconception that symptoms only happen when hormone is lost, when we know the symptoms start as hormone levels start to fluctuate. However, given that MHT is not yet widely familiar, I'll stick with HRT here.

in your blood. The idea of HRT is to replace your decreased or lost hormones with lab-made hormones. HRT is a combination of one, two or all three of the main ovarian hormones: oestrogen (always), progestagen (usually) and testosterone (sometimes). You take them to balance and supplement your natural hormone levels and you can access them as tablets or patches, gels, sprays or vaginal pessaries. What you require, what is safest for you, how you might prefer to use it and what it may cost will all be taken into account when choosing your best HRT option.

What about risks?

Yes, there are risks with taking HRT, but thankfully for almost all people under sixty years of age they are rare and, in general, the benefit of using HRT outweighs those risks. I'll go into detail on the risks as we go along.

The hormones – or what you are taking

HRT involves a cocktail of some or all three of the sex hormones: oestrogen, progestagen, testosterone. What people often don't realize, until they come to discuss it, is that HRT is usually taken as separate medications. It's not a single pill that you pop – like the combined contraceptive pill – it's a mix of different medications that give you a full and balanced HRT dose. Although, there is one pill that contains a weak combination of oestrogen, progestagen and testosterone – it's called Livial (or tibolone). It is a good triple hormone in that a single tablet gives a daily supply of the three hormones, but it is weak and it is taken orally, so must be confined to women at low risk of clots. Livial is useful for slim, non-smoking women whose periods are over and who want a little symptom relief. It is considered great for bones, too.

I can tell you what my HRT looks like, as an illustration of a typical set-up: I wear a patch and change it every Monday and Thursday, and that delivers my oestrogen. I swallow a Utrogestan gel cap (capsule pill) every night before bed, and that delivers my progestagen – and helps me sleep, too! I don't use testosterone, but if I did, I would do as most women do and apply a garden-pea-sized blob of gel to my inner thigh every day. Many other women prefer to use a patch called

Evorel Conti, which has both a bio-identical oestrogen (see Chapter 14) and a synthetic progestagen. They change the patch twice a week, job done for about €20 per month.

So that's the first thing to know about the HRT hormones – you'll be taking different types in different ways at different times and days. It sounds tedious, but you soon get used to it. While some of the products involved are costly, they are usually covered by the Irish Medical Card and Drugs Payment schemes.

Oestrogen, the main female sex hormone

Oestrogen is the main female sex hormone and the key hormone of HRT. It is produced mainly in the ovaries and is essential for a normal menstrual cycle, puberty and reproduction. It also has many non-reproductive effects in that it helps maintain cardiovascular, brain and bone health and is crucial for the integrity of collagen production and maintenance. There are various molecular forms of oestrogen found in the female body released by the human ovary, including:

- **E1 (estrone)**: the main hormone in the blood after your last period (which is why I think of it as old lady oestrogen – it's oestrogen for the over sixty-fives!)
- **E2 (estradiol)**: the main oestrogen in the blood in fertile women and the one used in most HRT combinations
- **E3 (estriol)**: made in the body of a foetus, so mainly found in the blood of pregnant women.

Do I take oral or non-oral oestrogen?

Some types of oestrogen are available in patches, gels, sprays and creams, while others come in tablet form. There are also local oestrogen products that are designed not to increase the blood levels of oestrogen, but only to work locally – this is vaginal oestrogen. Recently, bloodstream oestrogen delivery products that you wear in your vagina have become available in the UK and elsewhere. In other countries there are even more options. For example, in the USA there is a vaginal ring called Femring that delivers oestrogen to the blood through the vagina, but we don't have that in Ireland yet.

Tablet oestrogen is generally cheaper to buy, and most Irish pharmacies will have them in stock. However, when sex hormones are swallowed, they go through the liver and undergo what is known as the 'first pass effect' before they reach the main blood supply. This means that oral oestrogen is metabolized, or processed, in the liver before it works on our tissues. This first pass effect can be linked to more HRT-related side effects and risks than oestrogen that is delivered directly through the skin or vagina and into the main blood supply. Avoiding first pass metabolism by taking non-oral HRT is often beneficial because it:

- avoids non-absorption in people with gastro-intestinal absorption problems
- does not alter coagulation factors and therefore is not linked to an increased risk of blood clots (thrombosis) or stroke
- can lower triglycerides – oral oestrogen tends to increase them
- does not increase blood pressure
- has less impact on blood sugar and thyroid hormones
- may have less impact in terms of headache and migraine.

But for most women who are otherwise fit and well, oral oestrogen may be a convenient, inexpensive and safe choice.

Progestagen, protecting your womb-lining

HRT oestrogen must never be used for any length of time without some other hormone to balance its effects and to prevent womb-lining development, and this balance is usually provided by a progestagen. Progestagen is the collective term for all forms of the molecules, natural and synthetic, that affect the progesterone receptors in the body. The bio-identical progestagen, which is called progesterone, is an ovarian hormone that plays a key role in the menstrual cycle and period regulation, not to mention its big job – supporting pregnancy.

The progestagen's main function in HRT is to protect the lining of the womb from the effects of the HRT oestrogen. Left unchecked, oestrogen used on its own can cause thickening of the lining, as it would in preparation for pregnancy. But these womb-lining cell changes could lead to cancer. This is what happened when women in the USA in the 1970s took oestrogen on its own – it was later realized that they had much higher rates of womb-lining cancer. Now that we know this, it would be indefensible to prescribe oestrogen alone – unless you have had a hysterectomy. If you have had a hysterectomy and therefore do not have a womb, you usually do not take any progestagen – although that's not a hard and fast rule either. We want the womb-lining to remain stable and thin, and that is the progestagen's essential job when you take it as part of your HRT cocktail.

Which progestagen do I use and how do I take it?

Progestagens are available in many forms. Some are blended together with an oestrogen in patches, others come as tablets that can be swallowed or inserted vaginally, while many people use the progestagen-bearing intrauterine device (IUD or coil) known as Mirena for the progestagen element of their HRT.

How you choose to blend in the progestagen, when you take it and for how many days each month will all depend on where you are in your own cycles, your age, your desire for pregnancy, and other health issues that you can talk through with your GP.

Some progestagens control womb-lining thickness really well but are linked to more side effects. Others are less powerful at controlling the womb-lining but might be more tolerable. For example, people with depression, loss of concentration, brain fog and low libido should probably avoid the progestagens that are derived from androgens (for example, you'll see names like norethisterone (NET), levonorgestrel (LNG), desogestrel and dienogest) as they may make those symptoms worse. However, if you bleed heavily or too much, you may need those stronger, androgen-derived progestagens to deliver a manageable bleed. This is where the bit of witchcraft comes in – figuring out types and doses!

Price can be a problem with HRT for some people, although almost all forms of it are covered by the Medical Card and Drugs Payment schemes. Most HRT products use synthetic progestagen (a synthetic progestagen is also known as a progestin), and while very effective at protecting the womb-lining and usually very affordable, a progestin might give rise to more side effects for some people.

Micronized progesterone is often offered as part of the HRT cocktail. Micronization literally means to make smaller. The progesterone molecule is too large to be absorbed into the human bloodstream in its natural form, therefore it needs to be micronized down in a lab so that we can absorb it in a medicine. It is a natural, gentler and bio-identical progestagen. It is thought to be less likely to have a negative impact on the cardiovascular system, as well as being less likely to cause progestagen-related side effects, such as bloating and headache, but this is very subjective.

I described progestins as 'synthetic' above but, to be fair, all HRT is made in a factory/lab, but some hormones are molecularly identical to the ovary hormone they are replacing, while others are not. The molecularly identical products are called body-identical or bio-identical hormones – see Chapter 14 for more on those.

Do I take the progestagen every day or only for some days each month?

HRT cocktails are usually blended or tailored in such a way as to either make you bleed or continue to keep you not bleeding, depending on how you use the progestagen. There are pretty strict guidelines laid down by the BMS and NICE about when to use a 'period-creating' blend of oestrogen and progestagen versus when to use a 'no period' blend of oestrogen and progestagen. Sadly, you can't pick and choose. HRT will not 'turn off' your menstrual cycle, so if you have been having periods in the last year or two, you will probably be better off on a 'period-creating' blend of HRT. If you were to try a 'no period' blend of HRT and your own ovaries were still able to cause periods, you could get really heavy and unpredictable bleeding, which we always aim to avoid.

Period-creating HRT blends are also known as *cyclical HRT* aka *sequential HRT*. This involves taking oestrogen all the time, every day of the year, no breaks, but using progestagen for only ten to fourteen days per month. The withdrawal of the progestagen during the days you don't take it allows the womb-lining to shed. If there's anything built up in there, you will bleed.

No period HRT blends are also known as *continuous HRT*. This involves taking oestrogen all the time, no breaks, while also using progestagen all the time, every day, no breaks. If your womb-lining is thin and dormant, which is diagnosed as such by having had no periods for twelve months and being over fifty, then taking the progestagen in this way should not allow any bleeding and you should remain period-free. People on this blend may bleed when they first start their HRT, but it should settle on its own or, if necessary, with the addition of extra progestagen or a stronger progestagen (or even a Mirena coil).

Oestrogen makes the womb-lining thicker and more prone to bleeding, but the progestagen blocks that to an extent. You also have your own oestrogen and progestagen floating around your body from your ovaries. The rules are:

- if you have a womb and you need oestrogen and progestagen, and if you have not had a natural period in the last twelve months and you are over fifty years of age, the chances are your ovaries are not making eggs or periods any more and therefore you can try a no period HRT combination (the oestrogen and progestagen are used continuously)
  BUT
- if you have had a bleed in the last year or so, chances are your ovaries are not done just yet and therefore you need to use your oestrogen all the time, but you take the progestagen in a cyclical fashion – usually 2 weeks on/2 weeks off – and this makes you bleed every month.

You, as the patient, do not choose the regime – we, the doctor or health-care provider, do that. Our goal in designing your HRT is to make sure we do not cause heavy or unpredictable bleeding that may scare you and possibly lead to a series of unnecessary scans and referrals to the gynae clinic.

Testosterone, just as important for women as men

Testosterone is another important ovarian hormone for females. It plays a role in sexual desire and arousal, in the strength of your bones and in cognitive ability. Some of the testosterone found in the bloodstream of females comes from their ovaries and some from their adrenal glands, which sit above the kidneys. Testosterone decline is more likely to cause significant symptoms in younger people with POI and is particularly problematic when the ovaries are surgically removed (oophorectomy). This is because testosterone levels are much higher in women under thirty-five than in women over thirty-five – they decline naturally with aging – so to lose your ovarian testosterone overnight can put your libido into a tailspin. But this can also still happen to older women in the typical age range of menopause, between forty-five and fifty-five.

Testosterone HRT is available as a cream that is imported from Australia. It can be very costly, so many doctors are happy to prescribe a testosterone gel that is normally meant to be prescribed for male patients. (Using a medicine that is designed for something else is known as an 'unlicensed use of a licensed medical product'.) Whenever I am prescribing it, I warn the menopausal female patients to use the male testosterone gel in tiny doses. Testosterone is only licensed for hypoactive sexual desire disorder (HSDD), i.e. low libido, but we find it can help with many other symptoms as well, especially cognitive decline, joint pain and exercise tolerance. Scientific evidence is lacking here, though.

When used in the correct amounts, testosterone is unlikely to cause side effects. However, when used incorrectly, testosterone hormone can cause excessive body hair growth, thinning scalp hair, enlargement of the clitoris, and vocal cord changes. This is why we recommend that HRT testosterone users have their blood checked at least annually to monitor levels. We usually check levels after the first three months of use, and now some medical authorities even recommend getting your testosterone levels checked before you start the treatment. That's a question to put to your doctor when discussing your treatment plan.

Extra help for your vagina

We looked at local vaginal oestrogen in Chapter 6, as part of the discussion on the effect of menopause on the vagina. As explained there, the symptoms that can occur in the lower urinary and vaginal areas are known as GSM – genito-urinary syndrome of the menopause. The decline in the number of blood vessels that supply the uro-genital tract can result in hormone deficiency symptoms in the vulva, changes in the vaginal wall, changes in the bladder and pelvic floor. It is not unusual for menopausal patients to be affected by a dry, thin, less lubricated and uncomfortable vagina, and the problem is that not everyone on the usual systemic HRT (patches, pills, sprays and gels) will find it improves those symptoms. But what does work on those symptoms is low-dose, local vaginal oestrogen – applied right on the spot where you need it most.

This is available as a small pellet on a dispenser (E2, estradiol), or as a cream, or in a waxy, vaginal pessary (E3, estriol). You can also buy a three-month ring that delivers local vaginal oestrogen, but it is not licensed in Ireland and needs to be ordered and imported from the UK. You can choose to use vaginal oestrogen on its own if you only have vaginal symptoms, but most people tend to use it along with their systemic HRT blend. It is not an 'overdose' to use both oral/patch/gel HRT and a vaginal oestrogen.

You may need quite a bit of vaginal oestrogen at first, to set things right and regain your vaginal health. This usually entails a daily dose for the first two to three weeks and then much lower doses can be used thereafter. As with all forms of HRT, many guidelines will say 'lowest effective dose for the shortest duration of time', but the time frame is decided by you, not by your doctor. It is not wise to stop and start local vaginal HRT because each time you restart it, you have to use large doses again, some of which will leak into your blood, albeit only briefly. So, say you have had breast cancer and you really do not want any oestrogen in your blood, the best way to use the vaginal oestrogen is to start off with a high dose for two to three weeks, then stay on a low maintenance dose indefinitely, because if you stop completely, you may well have to start from scratch again. You can safely remain on local vaginal oestrogen for as long as you need it.

Why were women and doctors afraid of HRT for twenty years?

Having explained the science behind HRT and its benefits (which I go into in more detail in the rest of Part II), I want to return to the reason for much of the fear surrounding HRT, which often persists to this day. It goes back to a 2002 American study and it's important that you know exactly what it is and why it became controversial – and why its results do not, in fact, present a reason to avoid HRT.

HRT had been popular in the USA and Europe from the early 1970s and users derived great benefit from it. That situation started to change after 2002 when an editorial from an American medical study was published in the *Journal of the American Medical Association* (*JAMA*).

The *JAMA* editorial suggested that there was a link between using HRT and finding breast cancer. The study was called the Women's Health Initiative (WHI) and it was commissioned by the US government to look at many different aspects of the health of older women. They were particularly keen to see what factors affected heart disease and cancer. The ladies who were included in the study were almost all over fifty-five, some were as old as seventy-nine (although the majority were in their early sixties), and they were all offered one of a selection of daily tablets to take.

This was the largest randomized controlled trial of its kind, so the information was promising to be very reliable.

Some ladies in the WHI study were offered real HRT – the brand chosen was called Prempro (which was never available in Ireland). It was made up of an equine oestrogen hormone (made from the urine of pregnant horses) and a strong, synthetic progestagen that is manufactured under the name Provera.

Some ladies in the study were taking plain equine oestrogen called Premarin (short for PREgnant MAREs' urINe), some were taking the Prempro combination of equine oestrogen and Provera, and some were offered an identical pill that had no hormones in it at all (the placebo).

In the first five years of the study there was no difference in breast cancer rates in the three groups at all, but after five years a slight increase was noticed in the number of breast cancers being found in the women on the combination of oestrogen and progestagen. No increases were seen at all in the group on the plain oestrogen or in the placebo group.

In part, these increases may have been to do with the goals of the WHI group. The study was hoping to learn if older, sometimes unhealthy women would benefit from the reintroduction of female hormone in the form of HRT. There were some aspects of the WHI study that made it less relevant to the typical people we see in the GP surgery today. The criticisms of the WHI include:

- the exclusion of women with menopause symptoms
- the exclusion of women under fifty years of age
- the advanced age of the participants (average age sixty-two, but some were nearly eighty)
- the high rates of 'unblinding' (> 40 per cent of the participants were told whether they were using hormones or a placebo)
- the high rates of discontinuation (quitting the trial) in both groups and also a high crossover rate (asking to be moved over to the other group and therefore stop taking the medication)
- the use of a single, strong, oral HRT product.

There has also been criticism for the way in which the WHI data were reported. The *JAMA* editorial that followed the initial publication of the results referred to the association between HRT and breast cancer as 'markedly increased', although in fact the WHI authors reported a small relative risk that 'failed to reach statistical significance'. The *JAMA* team released this alarming interpretation to the main media before giving some of their own authors a chance to edit it, and without giving the wider medical community a chance to read, review and critique the data. In fact, the extra numbers of breast cancers diagnosed in the oestrogen + progestagen group were small.

Normally, the number of women who are diagnosed with breast cancer on a screening mammogram (this is for women who are over 50 in Ireland) is about 23 ladies (age group 50–59) for every 1,000 mammograms done. The WHI study found an additional four ladies: a total of 27 breast cancers when they did the 1,000 mammograms on the ladies who were taking the equine oestrogen and the Provera for more than five years.

This increase in detection was so small that it was not statistically significant. The figures were much lower than the extra number of breast cancers found in women who are overweight (47 cancers for every 1,000 mammograms). Moreover, there was no suggestion that the HRT was creating new cancers.

The WHI study did not suggest or prove that HRT caused breast cancers, only that there was a slight association in some older women over time.

Importantly, the women in the WHI study were not in any way representative of your typical perimenopausal/recently menopausal woman. No one with menopause symptoms was allowed in the study, some of the participants had already been diagnosed with serious medical conditions, such as heart disease, and no one was offered trans-dermal bio-identical oestrogen or one of the healthier progestagens.

The popular panic over HRT

Sadly, after the publication of the results in *JAMA*, things took an unfortunate turn. The popular papers then picked up the story and we started seeing terrifying headlines saying 'HRT causes breast cancer' – without any actual science to support this. It was so sad for Irish patients during those years. Hundreds of Irish women, as well as millions of women in the USA and Europe, stopped their HRT abruptly. Some were fine, but some got their symptoms back over-night and suffered greatly. Many were too terrified to seek help. Even when they did ask for advice, they didn't know who to believe. No matter how much some doctors tried to reassure patients about the facts on HRT and breast cancer, there were just as many other doctors who hadn't read all the information and were still warning patients to avoid HRT. This still happens today with less experienced doctors, gynaecologists and other health-care providers.

Things stayed this way for decades until finally, in November 2015, an update from the UK started to repair the damage. The National Institute for Health and Care Excellence (known as NICE), which is in charge of making recommendations and writing guidelines for doc-tors and nurses, published a review of menopause care and HRT that confirmed what menopause doctors had been saying all along: if your

patient is suffering and needs HRT to control troublesome menopause symptoms, you should feel confident to prescribe appropriate
HRT and you should support them in their choice. NICE pointed
out that most people who need HRT are young (well under the age
of the women in the WHI study) and are probably only going to stay
on HRT for a few years. This has slowly started a growing confidence
among many doctors about menopause care and HRT, and we have
thankfully noticed an increasing number of patients willing to talk
about their symptoms and seek advice.

So, can there be serious side effects with HRT?

Yes, there can, but thankfully they are very rare. For the vast majority of symptomatic people under sixty years of age the risks of HRT
use are far outweighed by the benefits of use. However, there are some
serious side effects linked to some forms of HRT, and you need to
know about these.

Breast cancer diagnosis (but not mortality) was found to be slightly
more common in people on oestrogen plus progestagen HRT if it
was used for more than four or five years (see the Women's Health
Initiative (WHI) study, described earlier in this chapter). The numbers are reassuringly low, however, and are similar to the number of
extra breast cancers found in women who drink more than two units
of alcohol a day. (I'll discuss breast cancer and the menopause in detail
in Chapter 18.)

The risks of *cardiovascular* (heart) and *cerebrovascular* (blood flow in the
brain) disease can be reduced in people on HRT who start taking it at
a young age, i.e. before the age of sixty. If you start HRT, particularly oral oestrogen HRT, more than ten years after your last period
and you are over sixty when you start taking it, then there may be an
increase in oestrogen-associated thrombosis, which can lead to heart
attack and stroke. We do not believe the risk is high if you try non-
oral oestrogen after sixty years of age, but we are advised to tread
more carefully as older women are more likely to have some vascular
disease already (see Chapter 17).

Diagnosis of *ovarian cancer* (certain types only) was found to be slightly higher in people taking HRT, with about one extra case of ovarian cancer for every 1,000 people on HRT.

The risk of *dementia* associated with hormone replacement therapy has delivered conflicting evidence. HRT is unlikely to increase the risk of dementia if you start it before the age of sixty, and there is some evidence to suggest it may protect against vascular dementia. Alzheimer's is dementia with no obvious cause, but vascular dementia we know to be caused by multiple mini-strokes, and this might be prevented if you start HRT early and use a non-oral oestrogen.

Common side effects of HRT

We use hormone replacement therapy to relieve the symptoms of perimenopause and make us feel better, but it also brings lots of proven health benefits. On the flip side, there are also potential side effects from each of the hormones, and particularly from oestrogen. Some of these are rare but serious, like blood clots. When you start taking any new medication you can experience side effects, and that's the case here, too. I will go through the serious and minor side effects that can come with your HRT in the chapters that follow.

For prescribers, the challenge is often figuring out which one of the hormones is causing the problem because there is a lot of overlap, and it can require a bit of detective work. To make matters even more complex, oestrogens and progestagens and androgens can all convert from one to another in different parts of our body. Head-wrecking!

Then there is also the possibility that HRT is unconnected to the symptom(s) you are experiencing. Not everything that happens to you when you use HRT comes from the HRT – although it does make sense to check that first and rule it in or out. If I had a nickel for every time someone on HRT attended the GP surgery or the ED with a symptom that they were told was probably the hormones but, when investigated, turned out to be something entirely different, I'd have a great big pile of nickels, I can tell you. It is human nature to be wary of new things, especially new medicines, which is not helped by the fact that there is also so much drama attached to being 'on hormones', like you have some kind of radioactive material inside of you, for crying out loud.

What you and your doctor and your pharmacist and everyone else need to remember is: *people with ovaries are supposed to have large amounts of sex hormones in their blood*, until they get to around the age of fifty-two to fifty-five. By then the levels will be much lower for most of us. Taking high-quality HRT under the age of, say, fifty-five years, for argument's sake, does not add anything to your system so much as it balances what is already in there. So, to scapegoat HRT for any and all health issues that arise while you are on it is usually a waste of time.

The chapters that follow here should help you to identify symptoms and sort the serious from the minor – including those that have got nothing to do with your HRT. I'm going to work through each hormone in turn – oestrogen, progestagen, testosterone and also local vaginal oestrogen – checking the benefits, minor side effects and serious side effects – all of which should give you a thorough working knowledge of the HRT cocktail and a better ability to weigh up what treatment would be best for you.

KEY TAKEAWAYS

- HRT use in women under sixty who need it is extremely safe: you have these hormones in your body already – we are just balancing them for you.
- Getting the right product for the right woman is an art form, and your GP may need to be very creative and be willing to think outside the box – so an experienced, knowledgeable GP is key.
- Most HRT side effects can be improved, but anxiety about being on HRT at all is something only you can control yourself.
- I know as much as most experts, and I use HRT without hesitation.

10. Oestrogen – the caped superhero!

Oestrogen decline happens naturally with aging. After your last period, loss of oestrogen impairs connective tissue metabolism in the bone, skin, discs in your back and other parts of your body. This can result in joint aches and pains and poor exercise tolerance. But one of the benefits of taking oestrogen HRT is that it has a protective effect against connective tissue loss, and could even reverse this process. In terms of perimenopause symptoms, oestrogen is a bit of a caped superhero. It comes with a long list of benefits and definitely makes us feel better.

Proven benefits of oestrogen

There is a long list of proven benefits:

- reduces flushes and sweats
- improves sleep, mood and memory
- helps prevent osteoporosis and fractures at all areas of the body
- reduces the risk of getting Type 2 diabetes
- prevents glaucoma in the eyes
- reverses collagen loss, therefore can help with joint and pelvic floor issues, like urine leakage
- improves the loss of muscle mass commonly seen in older people
- delays/prevents heart attacks and heart muscle failure
- decreases 'bad' LDL cholesterol and increases 'good' HDL cholesterol.

Suspected benefits of oestrogen (not yet scientifically proven)

There are a number of suspected benefits:

- prevents certain types of dementia as well as Parkinson's disease
- prevents macular degeneration in the eye, which is a common cause of vision loss in older people
- keeps teeth and gums healthier and helps prevent old age tooth loss
- protects against colorectal cancer.

So, what's not to like about oestrogen? As you know, my patch and I will never be parted, so I'm a convert. But that said, it does have the potential for side effects and more serious harm, which, while posing only a small risk, most certainly needs to be discussed.

The side effects and risks of oestrogen as found in HRT can be divided into major (i.e. serious or life-threatening) and minor. I've never liked the word 'minor' in medicine because a non-life-threatening side effect can still have a major impact on your life. So how about, for our purposes, we divide them into dangerous versus not dangerous.

Non-dangerous but annoying side effects of HRT oestrogen

You may experience any of the following:

- nausea
- breast discomfort/swelling
- womb-lining stimulation (and possible unexpected vaginal bleeding)
- leg cramps
- headache
- fluid retention/ bloating
- reaction/allergy to adhesive or gel (not a reaction to the actual medicine, but to things like the pasty stuff that a tablet is

made up of – that might contain soya, for example, which is a problem if you're allergic to soya)
- heartburn/indigestion.

Fixes for non-dangerous oestrogen side effects

There are a number of potential fixes for these side effects:

1. consider lowering the overall dose
2. consider changing the route of administration
3. consider the pros and cons of steady release (i.e. constant) versus pulsatile delivery (i.e. the hormone is released in bursts, with breaks in between).

Let's now take a look at each of these in turn.

FIX 1: LOWER THE OVERALL DOSE

The usual 'dose' of oestrogen in most HRT products is 50mcg a day – this is the dose that we usually start you off with. Some women need much more than 50mcg daily, especially the POI ladies. Other women can get by with less, that's usually the older ladies. The books all say use the lowest *effective* dose, so we may have to try different amounts to get the right response for you.

The amount of oestrogen you need to use in your HRT for health protection is actually very low. As little as a 25mcg patch or 1–2 daily pumps of gel or 1 spray a day or a 1mg daily tablet of oestrogen will protect your bones and your heart and your brain, but you may need more than that for menopause symptom control. Plus, the younger you are, chances are the more you will need. But with the use of greater amounts of oestrogen comes the risk of more side effects.

The key is to achieve the right balance, and that will be a collaboration between you (the user) and us (the prescribers). It is usually smart to start with a lower dose first, so as not to overwhelm your body, which might be quite oestrogen deprived, and thereby avoid kicking off side effects. 'Start slow and low' is my advice to colleagues and patients, especially if you have had oestrogen-related health complaints in the past. For example, if you are a known headache sufferer and if you found your headaches got worse when you were taking the contraceptive pill or when you were pregnant, then guess what? HRT may well start up some headache activity, too. But if we tiptoe into it, instead of lashing it on in spades, then hopefully your brain will play ball and the headaches, or other symptoms, won't return. You do need to be prepared for this, however, and for the other non-dangerous side effects of HRT, because it can take a few weeks of feeling yuk before all the side effects resolve and you get all the benefit without the hassle. Easier said than done, I know!

Nausea is probably the easiest side effect to tackle effectively. If you are on a daily oral pill, take it with food to help with the nausea. And if the current dose is too much for you, go lower until the nausea settles. If this doesn't help, you can try a non-oral oestrogen, but this will not necessarily fix the problem either.

Breast discomfort/pain – well, obviously let's make sure you don't feel a lump and that you have regular mammograms, if you are eligible. Also remember that breast pain is a very unusual way to detect breast cancer. The most common sign of breast cancer is a lump, nipple changes or something showing up on a mammogram. Breast pain is often nothing to do with cancer, but it can be persistent, uncomfortable and worrying. Cause and effect can be far apart in time as well. I still get an ache in my left boob in the area where I had mastitis in 1990, thanks to the endless breastfeeding my big lad inflicted on me (*thanks, Mur!*). If you do experience breast pain, lowering the dose of oestrogen may help, and a good supportive bra is also essential. I recommend a soft sports bra in bed at night for breast pain sufferers. Also try a big cabbage leaf poultice between your bra and your breast when you sleep. This is the old wives' tale cure for mastitis, but it can't hurt for 'normal' breast pain and may help.

Bloating is a nightmare – as most of us already know – and it is the curse of ovarian hormones. I wake up each morning with a flattish gut, but by bedtime I have a beer belly, and I don't drink beer. The science of bloating is complex, but there are some recommendations for people with severe bloating/fluid retention, such as taking gamma linoleic supplements, which you find in evening primrose or starflower oils. I'm not sure how much science supports that, but it's a common recommendation.

Keeping hydrated is also helpful. You'd think too much water would make you retain more fluid, but the opposite seems to be the case. Also, avoiding too much salt – and that means processed foods as well. And, most importantly, regular exercise. Physical movement helps blood return from your feet to your heart and can be an aid to reducing bloating. You can also try lowering your dose of oestrogen, which can help, as can changing the progestagen. Progestagen choices in Ireland for HRT include: micronized progesterone (brand name Utrogestan) or dydrogesterone (brand name Duphaston) or norethis-terone (brand name Noriday) or levonorgestrel (brand name Mirena) or medroxyprogesterone acetate (brand name Provera). See Chapter 11 for more information on this.

FIX 2: CHANGE THE ROUTE OF ADMINISTRATION

Oestrogen can be taken in a tablet on its own, in a tablet with a proges-tagen included, in a patch, in a gel, or in a spray. Using oral oestrogen is more likely to cause non-dangerous side effects like nausea, headache and heartburn, so, logically, if you are getting HRT-related nausea or headache or heartburn, you could try the non-oral delivery route instead. Alternatively, if you are experiencing an irritation or an aller-gic reaction to your oestrogen gel or patch, you might try a pill or a spray instead. It's about monitoring your own body and reactions and going back to the doctor as and when you need to, to discuss what you are feeling and what your options are to deal with it.

FIX 3: CONSIDER THE PROS AND CONS
OF STEADY RELEASE VERSUS PULSATILE DELIVERY

When you are having regular menstrual periods, oestrogen release from the ovaries does not usually change too much over the course of a given day – although you will have more or less oestrogen in some days of the month than others. Conversely, progesterone levels do seem to follow circadian or ultradian rhythms – progesterone can rise or fall in as little as 90 minutes (ultradian) and will certainly change over any specific 24-hour day (circadian).

Oestrogen blood levels do not always reflect what is going on in your cells, though, and certainly not how you feel. We know some patients who have very low blood levels of oestrogen feel fine in some cases, while other people with very high blood levels of oestrogen are still struggling with symptoms. So prescribing hormone therapy is not always as easy as saying, 'Here's some oestrogen, all will be grand now, goodbye.'

There are some side effects that seem to respond to whether you are using oestrogen in a steady release, 24-hour-a-day regime or just taking doses of it in a pulsatile regime. When you wear a patch, estradiol is dripping into your blood all the time, day and night, and this may be good for alleviating some non-dangerous side effects, such as headache, but could make issues like sore breasts or bloating worse. So, if you are on a patch and experiencing symptoms, try a gel or spray as they do not deliver oestrogen in a steady, continuous release. If you are on a spray or gel already, try a patch.

Possible dangerous side effects of HRT oestrogen

These are rare potential side effects, but we need to talk about:

- breast/endometrial/ovarian cancer
- blood clots
- stroke.

Breast cancer

As I explained in the previous chapter, women who are in their forties and fifties grew up with the widespread belief that HRT causes breast cancer. This was, as we know, based on the parameters and interpretation of the results of the WHI trial. We know this is not true. HRT oestrogen is not a carcinogen, which means it does not cause breast cancer. However, it stands to reason that if you already have the beginnings of an oestrogen-sensitive breast cancer, then adding in extra oestrogen may accelerate the development of the disease. Progestagen also plays a role, and newer small-scale studies all seem to point the finger at the progestagen in HRT as the probable culprit for that small additional risk of breast cancer – the suggestion being that MPA (which was the progestagen used in the WHI study) may in fact be the form of progestagen that is most likely to increase breast cancer diagnosis rates. Whereas micronized progesterone (P4) and dydrogesterone are the forms of progesterone that are least likely to increase breast cancer rates. However, it must be noted that none of this is definitive as of yet, and lots more information is needed before we can give exact details when it comes to HRT and breast cancer.

Endometrial (womb-lining) cancer

This is very rare when HRT is used correctly. When HRT was being developed in the 1960s and 1970s, doctors frequently just provided patients with some oestrogen, no blending or balancing. We call this 'unopposed' oestrogen use. After a few years, patients were turning up with abnormal bleeding, and the link between using plain oestrogen and developing womb-lining cancer was discovered. A Cochrane* review showed that the risks associated with unopposed oestrogen replacement are both dose- and duration-dependent, with exposure between one and three years.

In the last forty years we have become acutely aware of the dangers of using unopposed oestrogen for HRT. It is never recommended. Even if you have had an ablation (removal of most of the womb-lining), you need the HRT progestagen alongside oestrogen. Even if you are on the mini contraceptive pill (or POP), which contains progestagen, you still need the HRT progestagen because the POP progestagens are too weak.

The correct use of an approved HRT progestagen delivers enormous protection from abnormalities of the womb-lining that might have occurred if you were taking oestrogen on its own. It is so effective

* The Cochrane library (previously known as the Cochrane Collaboration) is a British international charitable organization formed to organize medical research findings to facilitate evidence-based choices about health interventions involving health professionals, patients and policy makers. It includes 53 review groups that are based at research institutions worldwide. Cochrane has approximately 30,000 volunteer experts from around the world. All doctors know the Cochrane group.

at safeguarding your womb-lining that people like me – older women who use a low dose of progestagen every single day (which is okay if you are no longer getting natural periods) – have a lower lifetime risk of womb-lining cancer than women who do not take HRT. Patients who use HRT where the progestagen is given every day (the 'no period' way) have a lower risk of womb-lining cancer than people who never took HRT. So long as you are getting your HRT from someone who knows the rules, you are safe. We can only use certain progestagens at specific doses when we offer HRT – this is because these progestagens have been studied to make sure they will prevent womb-lining build-up and not allow the oestrogen in your HRT to increase your risk of womb-lining cancer. (See Chapter II for detailed information on progestagens and HRT.)

Ovarian cancer

There may be a slight increase in the risk of developing ovarian cancer associated with HRT use. However, this risk is small and should be taken in the context of the overall benefits it affords to the patient. (Weirdly, studies have shown that using the strong doses of oestrogen and progestagen as found in the contraceptive pill protects you against ovarian cancer if you use it when you are younger. Nothing is straightforward, is it?)

Blood clots

This risk is only seen with oral oestrogen. Oestrogen affects the clotting proteins that help prevent haemorrhage. There may be advantages to that in some situations, for example, having sticky, clotty blood protects pregnant women from bleeding to death in childbirth. However, venous thromboembolism (VTE) is a dangerous and potentially life-threatening disease that causes little chunks of blood cells (a clot or thrombus) to gather in one of the deep veins.

This is not to be confused with a bruise or varicose veins. If you bump into something hard, you might damage the surface or 'superficial' veins under your skin and in your muscle and end up with a bruise. If you have inherited weak valves in your superficial veins, you might end up with swollen, gnarly veins at the back of your calves. These are called 'varicosities' and can be a problem. Not only do they look unpleasant but if you were to injure them and they started bleeding, they might not stop for a long time. These vein conditions are completely different from the blockage of one of the deep veins buried within the deeper tissues in your body.

Many studies on HRT have shown an increased risk of VTE, especially in the first year or so after starting HRT. Thankfully, there is excellent evidence to show that this risk is confined to oral oestrogen and that the use of transdermal (TD – meaning via the skin, as with a patch) oestrogen in average doses will not increase your risk of VTE. This also goes for women who already have increased risk of clotting problems (thrombophilias).

Stroke and heart attack

The risk of **stroke** is age-related and overall the risk is low in women under the age of sixty. Oral estradiol is likely to be associated with a small increase in the risk of stroke. This is likely to be dose-related, therefore the lowest effective dose should be prescribed, or else use transdermal estradiol, which is unlikely to increase the risk of stroke above your own baseline risk.

Transdermal oestrogen is advisable for people with risk factors and people over the age of sixty. If you are at risk of stroke, the type of progesterone used in HRT may have an effect on the level of risk posed to you. For this reason, try micronized progesterone or the dydrogesterone progestagens, in combination with transdermal estradiol.

What are the differences between the various HRT oestrogens and their risks?

In the earliest HRT products, the most popular oestrogen used was conjugated equine oestrogen (CEE), derived from the urine of pregnant mares. CEE is a cocktail of horse hormone so complex and strong that it always amazes me that it didn't cause *more* harm. It was the only form of HRT oestrogen studied in the large WHI trial (see Chapter 9) which, flawed as it was, provided a baseline of data that we use to inform patients to this day. It is still one of the most commonly prescribed forms of HRT oestrogen in the world today, possibly because it is cheap.

I don't think I'd like the idea of equine molecules running around my body. As a result, I almost never prescribe, or even mention, CEE to patients! Some of the molecules are known to cause chemical reactions in the liver and are therefore likely to increase your risk of VTE. Some have been linked to bad outcomes with regard to heart attack, blood clots, stroke, et cetera.

To reiterate: most of the data we have on HRT and disease prevention comes from clinical trials that used CEE as the oestrogen in their HRT, so it's not an accurate reflection of today's HRT landscape. Since then, other forms of oestrogen HRT have come to market, including oral estradiol (E2), transdermal 17 beta estradiol (body-identical E2) and, most recently, foetal liver oestrogen which is promised to be one of the safest oestrogens around. It has recently been released in Europe and the USA in a contraceptive pill. We'll have to see if it lives up to its promise.

KEY TAKEAWAYS

- The oestrogen we naturally produce in our bodies brings a range of health benefits. It's a necessary hormone for the maintenance of good female health, which is why we feel symptoms when the level of oestrogen fluctuates and falls away. This is why we use HRT – to balance our oestrogen levels.

- Not everything that goes wrong in your middle life can be fixed by HRT. It is not a panacea, but HRT is by far the most effective way to control perimenopause and menopause symptoms.

- HRT is not the choice of every person, and it's not suitable for every person, but it is safe and effective for almost everyone who chooses to use it. (I'm saying 'almost' because there are some medical conditions and treatments that might preclude its use.)

- HRT is a blend of hormones, and that blend must fit your specific needs and circumstances. There is patience required as you and your doctor figure out exactly what will work best for you.

11. Progestagen – the yin to oestrogen's yang

There can be progestagen-related minor, non-dangerous side effects, but I have never heard of a dangerous side effect from progestagen, especially from the low-dose natural stuff. You can never say never, but the data don't show any known dangerous side effects.

In terms of benefits, the first thing to say is that not all progestagens are the same. Different HRT products contain many different progestagens. These are the progestagens for which there are good data and evidence to say they will protect your womb-lining against oestrogen. They are 'approved' for use in an HRT combo available in Ireland and the UK.*

- P4 micronized progesterone, which is sold under the trade name Utrogestan: can be used orally or intra-vaginally.
- Dydrogesterone, which is sold on its own under the trade name Duphaston. It is also available as a combination tablet with oestrogen in the products that go by the trade name Femoston. Dydrogesterone and P4 are both progesterone derivatives, meaning they are less likely to cause androgenic (male hormone) side effects.
- Norethisterone acetate (NET) comes in many forms. It is available in a patch blended with oestrogen and sold under the trade name Evorel Conti. It can be sourced on its own as a pill with trade names like Primolut and Noriday. It is also available as a pill combined with oestrogen and comes under various trade names, such as Activelle, Trisequens and Kliogest.

* Assiduous Irish readers doing their own research may come across other progestagens not available in Ireland or the UK (for example, norethindrone acetate, norgestrel and dienogest).

- Medroxyprogesterone acetate is available on its own under the trade name Provera, or can be found blended with an oestrogen in a combination HRT called Indivina.
- Drospirenone is available on its own in the UK but not yet in Ireland – here, it's used in tablets with oestrogen in them called Angeliq. It is a spironolactone derivative. Spironolactone is a diuretic drug (encourages the body to shed liquid), therefore is claimed to be less likely to cause fluid retention and bloating as many other progestagens can do.
- Levonorgestrel (LNG) found in the 52mg IUCD (Mirena): intrauterine only – there are LNG pills but only available in the UK; we never use them in Ireland for HRT.

And let's not forget the unusual HRT option called tibolone, which is not an oestrogen and progesterone cocktail like all the rest, but a synthetic steroid molecule that, once passed through the liver, becomes activated into other molecules, known as metabolite molecules. These have weak but noticeable effects on oestrogen, progesterone and testosterone receptors on the body. This means tibolone is neither oestrogen nor progesterone nor testosterone, but a little bit of all three. It's sold under the trade name Livial in Ireland.

Benefits of progestagen

Your womb-lining is a very active place – the layers are constantly being built up and then shed, the cells within the lining change from one part of the month to the other, either preparing for a pregnancy or getting rid of last month's build-up to start afresh for this month's attempt. Progestagens protect the womb-lining by keeping it quiet and subdued.

We want your womb-lining to calm down and stay stable while you are on HRT, otherwise you may get heavy or unexpected bleeding, which can be an upsetting experience. So, progestagen is added to oestrogen in HRT to balance and 'oppose' the effects of oestrogen on the womb-lining. Oestrogen thickens and destabilizes the womb-lining; progestagen usually does the opposite. So, it's a yin and yang thing with oestrogen, giving you a safer balance of hormones. You

must not use oestrogen in the form of patches, sprays, gels or oral pills if you are not also using a progestagen. (It is okay to use vaginal oestrogen cream or pessaries on their own, though, as they do not expose the womb-lining to dangerous side effects.)

Apart from protecting your womb-lining some progestagens have been shown to have a range of benefits from protecting bone health to improving vasomotor symptoms (hot flushes) and reducing anxiety. Dr Jerilynn Prior, Professor of Endocrinology and Metabolism at the University of British Columbia, found that oral micronized progesterone (P4) is effective against hot flushes and night sweats, improves sleep and helps protect bones and heart. She has even suggested that P4 on its own is equally or more effective than HRT estradiol in improving cardiovascular function (more work is needed before P4 replaces the oestrogen in HRT, but it is a potentially exciting development).

I know for sure that many HRT users say they like some of the effects of progestagen. Some people have told me that they take their P4 last thing before bedtime and they get a great night's sleep as a result. That's purely anecdotal evidence – and of course it's dose- and user-dependent – but I've heard it enough to take notice. Although it only seems to work if you take it by mouth. Vaginal P4 does not do that first pass through the liver, and you seem to miss out on some of the sleepy effects if you use it internally rather than orally. For now, let's just say that if you have a womb and you use oestrogen, you must also take progestagen – and if it helps you sleep, all the better.

There are some situations where even women who have had their womb removed are also advised to use progestagen with their HRT oestrogen. One common situation is where a woman has had her womb removed in an effort to give relief from moderate to severe endometriosis (see Chapter 20). But even if you have no womb and no endometriosis risk, it would still be hard to rationalize taking P4 just for good sleeping patterns.

The WHI data tell us that it is as much the progestagen in HRT as it is the oestrogen – if not more so – that is linked to the small extra risk of breast cancer. In addition, many breast cancers have progestagen receptors on them, along with oestrogen receptors, so I would not be overly complacent about progestagen. It may give you symptom relief if used on its own without oestrogen, but I would not consider that 'safer' regarding breast cancer risk.

Non-dangerous but annoying side effects of HRT progestagen

You may experience any of the following:

- fluid retention
- PMS-type symptoms
- breast tenderness
- headaches
- depression and/or anxiety
- flatulence
- increased appetite
- acne
- backache
- lower abdominal pain.

Fixes for non-dangerous progestagen side effects

There are two potential approaches to fixing any side effects:

1. consider lowering the dose or potency, or
2. consider changing the delivery route.

FIX 1: LOWER THE DOSE OR POTENCY

Some progestagens are more potent than others. The long list of progestagens mentioned above all have individual potencies. Too much or too strong a progestagen for your body, and the more you might be inclined to experience non-dangerous side effects. P4 is considered the mildest progestagen, but that still doesn't mean it suits everybody.

Some people find the 200mg for two weeks a month dose is too much to deal with. Sometimes we can protect your womb-lining and minimize your side effects by giving less over a longer period (for example, 100mg taken for three weeks each month). Some people prefer the Mirena coil (see pages 158–9), which is meant to put less progestagen into the blood. However, there is plenty of evidence, backed up by patient testimonials, to say that the first six months of use is the time when you are most likely to experience the minor side effects, but if you can hold on, the remaining four and a half years should be fine.

There have been lots of studies that have examined micronized progesterone or P4. Some have shown that oral P4 provides endometrial protection if taken for twelve to fourteen days per month in a dose of 200mg/day for up to five years. Another study has shown that vaginal P4 may provide endometrial protection if used for ten days per month, or every other day, in a dose of 100mg per day for up to three to five years. Importantly, though, a systematic review concluded that *transdermal* micronized progesterone does not provide sufficient endometrial protection. This means you may not use micronized progesterone in a cream or a patch because it is not strong enough to protect your womb-lining. This is a serious issue as many 'compounded' bio-identical HRT products (see Chapter 14) put the micronized progesterone into a cream, even though we all know the safety data are poor for this practice.

Some people like the norethisterone (NET) progestagen on the patch that has the oestrogen and progestagen together. This is excellent for convenience. A combined HRT patch is also handy if you keep forgetting to take your progestagen. I often start people off on the only oestrogen/progestagen patch combo we have in Ireland – Evorel Conti – if they are new to the whole HRT thing. It is so simple to just apply the new patch twice a week, and away you go – nothing else for you to remember to do.

For purists, those who want entirely body-identical HRT, this will not be acceptable (as norethisterone is a potent artificial progestagen that is derived from an androgen), and they will need to use a transdermal oestrogen and the micronized progesterone tablet. That is my own cocktail of choice, but it takes commitment. I choose to take my micronized progesterone tablet at night, before going to bed. It costs me a bit more than using an Evorel Conti patch and is a bit fussier, but it is considered the safest/healthiest/best mix of HRT and it suits me – but this may not suit other people.

On the rare occasion that I run out of my own micronized

progesterone and I let a few days slide without it (I know – I am break-ing the rules!), I can sometimes start to bleed – and it can be heavy. It doesn't scare me. I know what I've done: I have taken the brakes off my womb-lining and this is not wise (so, don't you do it either!).

FIX 2: CHANGE THE DELIVERY ROUTE

You can sometimes get relief from non-dangerous progestagen side effects by delivering it in a different way. Bloating seems to improve for some people when they take their progestagen at night-time – as we usually do with P4 and dydrogesterone. Others prefer a steady, continual low dose, like you get with the oestrogen and progestagen combination patches, or even with a Mirena coil and some transder-mal oestrogen products.

As mentioned earlier, progesterone levels do rise and fall, follow-ing circadian (daily) or ultradian (hourly) rhythms. Progesterone also becomes progressively more abundant at the end of a monthly cycle (i.e. in the premenstrual phase). People are sometimes highly sensi-tive to the effects of progestagen and we can, very occasionally, bend the rules to protect your womb-lining as best we can while aiming to expose you to as little progestagen as possible. But I would not rec-ommend this unless you have exhausted all other options.

One approach is to take the least offensive progestagen on only ten to twelve days of every ten weeks. 'Long-cycle progestagen' regimes are mentioned in the British Menopause Society (BMS) handbook, but they do expose you to a slightly higher risk of womb-lining build-up and possible abnormal cell changes, so I would usually suggest getting a scan of the womb done once every year that you are doing this, particularly if you start bleeding heavily and persistently.

Fixes for specific side effects

There are a number of additional fixes we can try, targeted at specific side effects.

- **Fluid retention**: try a new progestagen or use P4 vaginally.
- **PMS-type symptoms**: try a new progestagen or use P4 vaginally.

- **Breast tenderness**: try a new progestagen or use P4 vaginally.
- **Headaches**: try a new progestagen.
- **Depression and/or anxiety**: try a new progestagen, try using a long-cycle regime.
- **Flatulence**: no ideas here – sorry!
- **Increased appetite**: try using night-time progestagen.
- **Acne**: change to an option that puts less progestagen or a more natural progestagen in the blood, such as Mirena or P4.
- **Backache**: try a new progestagen or use P4 vaginally.
- **Lower abdominal pain**: try a new progestagen or use P4 vaginally.

The BMS says that:

Progestogen side effects may be reduced by using natural progesterone in the form of oral capsules or transvaginal pessaries. Data from large observational studies have shown a lower risk of blood clots and breast cancer with micronized progesterone (P4) compared to that seen with synthetic progestogens.

Some progestagens appear to have a stronger impact on the body than others. The two safest progestagens are thought to be P4 or micronized progesterone (brand name Utrogestan) and dydrogesterone (brand name Duphaston). Blood clots and breast cancer rates were lowest among women using these compared with, say, the very popular Noriday and Provera. Only lately have we come to learn that certain very strong, very high-dose progestagens may promote blood clots, but none of these is used in HRT.

Symptoms of fluid retention result from the effects that certain progestagens have on the kidneys. Micronized progesterone has a more selective effect on progesterone receptors and results in less interaction in the kidneys. Recent evidence suggests that HRT regimens containing micronized progesterone can minimize the metabolic impact and side effects associated with other progestagens. For example, drospirenone, a newer progestin, which is used in contraception all the time, and is also available in an oral HRT called Angeliq.

It's also important to note that the levonorgestrel intrauterine system (Mirena) has a five-year licence in Ireland (four years in the

UK, but the BMS agrees that five years is acceptable) and it should also minimize progestagen side effects.

Dangerous side effects of HRT progestagen

I don't know of any real-life serious side effects of progestagen use because in thirty-five years of clinical work, I haven't met a single patient who suffered any, I'm glad to say. That said, it is recommended not to take progestagen if you have had or are currently receiving treatment for:

- breast cancer
- porphyria (an inherited blood disorder that puts you at risk of clotting problems)
- abnormal liver blood tests.

This is true for the oestrogen in HRT, too. Some cancers, particularly breast cancers, can have progestagen receptors on them, so we would not routinely prescribe oestrogen or progestagen to patients with breast cancer.

The biggest issue you are likely to meet with progestagen is tolerability (ensuring the side effects are minimal enough that you can get the benefits from a hormone without having to pay too high a price in side effects) and bleeding patterns. Unexpected or heavy, persistent bleeding is quite common at the beginning of HRT use (see Chapter 15). It can be frightening, but it is almost always caused by an imbalance between the dose and type of your progestagen and oestrogen.

How much do you need to take?

Obviously, you and your doctor will work together to determine the correct dosage for you, but in the interests of you understanding more about what your GP might prescribe, here is the *minimum* required dose of progestagen *for people who don't get periods any more* to keep bleeding under control.

- 100mg/day Utrogestan
- 5–10mg/day Duphaston
- 2.5mg/day Provera
- 1mg/day Noriday
- Mirena coil over 5 years

However, you might need more than the above doses to keep your womb-lining quiet, especially if it was causing problems before you ever went on HRT.

Here is the *minimum* monthly required dose of progestagen to keep bleeding under control *for people who still get periods*, even if they only come once in a while.

- 1mg/day x 10 days for Noriday
- 200mg/day x 12 days for Utrogestan
- 10mg/day x 10–14 days for Provera
- 10–20mg/day x 12 days for Duphaston
- Mirena coil over 5 years

As above, if your womb-lining was giving you trouble before you started on HRT, you might need more than these doses. If bleeding continues to be a problem, there are a few other options open to your doctor, including adding in a bleed-slowing medicine like tranexamic acid, or even referring you to a gynaecological service to have investigations and discuss treatments for bleeding problems.

KEY TAKEAWAYS

- Progestagen has been proven to be a very safe and effective ingredient of HRT.
- Progestagen is essential because you must balance the effects of the oestrogen you are taking and prevent it affecting your womb-lining.
- It can take time to find the right progestagen for your body. I often have to try several different types with a patient before we hit on the one she can tolerate. So be prepared to start on a progestagen and monitor how you're feeling – and then change it up if you need to.

12. Testosterone – the trusty sidekick

Testosterone and other androgens – male hormones – are just as important to female bodies as they are to male bodies. When we are young, under thirty-five years of age, our ovaries produce a wider selection of testosterone molecules than oestrogen molecules every day. The ovaries are not the only source of testosterone, with 50 per cent coming from the adrenal glands.

Most of the information we apply to using testosterone for female menopause symptoms comes from studies looking at people who experience early menopause, either due to POI or for medical reasons, where the drop in testosterone levels is likely to be extreme. This can cause lots of unwanted symptoms, the most common being reductions in sexual desire, arousal and ability to orgasm. But there are many other symptoms, too, including brain fog and joint aches, as well as exercise intolerance for some people. According to the British Menopause Society low testosterone has also been linked to fatigue, poor quality of life scores, low mood, headache, deterioration of bone and muscle mass (osteoporosis and sarcopaenia).

Testosterone use for menopausal women

Until recently, we did not usually measure your testosterone levels to decide if you needed testosterone in your HRT – we just listened to your symptoms. Clinics differed on this – some didn't measure beforehand, others did – and those who didn't were operating on the basis that it would be highly unlikely for a perimenopausal or menopausal woman to have *excess* testosterone in her blood. But this has changed recently, and the advice in 2022 is that a baseline test should be performed prior to use.

In my clinic, if you appear to have symptoms of low testosterone, we test your levels, then we try some testosterone for a few months and see what happens. This is called 'empirical therapy' – the medical version of 'suck it and see'. If you feel better, you keep using it. That said, there are some requirements for testosterone use that you must fulfil. We insist on getting blood levels once you start taking testosterone. Unlike oestrogen and progestagen levels in standard HRT, testosterone levels must be monitored to make sure you are not absorbing too much. After two to three months using testosterone, a blood test must be done to measure the amount of testosterone in the blood.★ You should get that test done every year or so when you are on testosterone therapy in order to prevent overuse.

In general, when we offer testosterone therapy to patients, we do it in conjunction with oestrogen and progestagen HRT, but the British Menopause Society (BMS) reassuringly says:

> Although the NICE NG23 guideline recommends that systemic HRT should be prescribed before a trial of testosterone, there are trial data in women with HSDD [low or no sex drive] which indicate that testosterone used without systemic oestrogen is equally effective and safe.

In other words: if you just want to try some testosterone first, without the other two hormones, you can do that.

The only caveat I have about the use of testosterone on its own is that an imbalance between testosterone versus oestrogen can result in side effects like acne and body hair, which we see in teens and sometimes in post-menopausal women who are not on HRT. This is because as an older woman ages, her body still makes testosterone but makes less and less oestrogen. That leads to testosterone imbalance, which leads to symptoms like unwanted hair growth – the bane of so many older women's lives!

It is possible that testosterone-related side effects could be more of an issue if your levels of oestrogen are fluctuating from day to day

---

★ Your level is calculated by measuring total testosterone (TT) as well as the levels of sex hormone-binding globulin (SHBG; this is a protein made by the liver that binds with sex hormones found in both women and men). You divide the TT by the SHGB and multiply by 100. That result ought to be < 5 per cent.

while your testosterone levels remain high. However, any side effects and risks are minimal and reversible if your blood levels of testosterone are kept within the normal female range. The message is to go easy on the T!

Benefits of testosterone therapy

There are a number of benefits associated with testosterone therapy.

- It is licensed for the treatment of low libido in menopause.
- It acts on dopamine levels in the blood to improve sexual functions like arousal and the ability to achieve orgasm, as well as improving mood in general.
- Some studies have shown benefits on the skeleton, cognition, well-being and the vagina.
- Testosterone maintains normal metabolic function and can help prevent you losing muscle mass.

Non-dangerous side effects of testosterone therapy

Note that these only occur with an *excess* of male hormone:

- increased body hair where you rub the gel
- body hair growth increase
- scalp hair loss, especially 'male pattern' hair loss
- acne and oily skin
- deepening of voice
- enlargement of the clitoris.

Fixes for testosterone side effects

Almost all side effects are reversible once you stop taking it, so at the first sign of any issue, just come off the testosterone, get your levels checked, and discuss with your doctor going back on it with slower frequency and lower dosage.

The following fixes should help specific side effects.

- **Hair growth or darkening at site of application**: spread the testosterone more thinly and change the place you rub it in, to one with less hair (such as back of the knee or inner thigh) and/ or use less of it or apply it less often.
- **Acne/oily skin**: use less of it or apply it less often, and maybe get a blood test done, to ascertain if you already have a high level of testosterone in your body.

Testosterone products you may be offered

Before I mention some products licensed for use in Ireland, please note they are all treatments you use on your skin. Oral testosterone is not appropriate for menopause symptom control in women as it has adverse effects on cholesterol, liver function and clotting factors.

AndroFeme 1

There is just one form of testosterone replacement that is licensed for use in menopausal women available in the Republic of Ireland. It is an Australian product that is available to order via your GP/pharmacy. It contains a 1 per cent testosterone cream in 50ml tubes with a replaceable screw cap. The usual dose of AndroFeme 1 is 0.5ml per day, and the cream must be applied every day. That means each tube should last just over three months and at about €100 to €120 a tube, that works out to be about €40 a month.

Testogel

This is a testosterone gel licensed for testosterone replacement in men, but it is an identical testosterone molecule to the testosterone in AndroFeme 1. It is also a 1 per cent testosterone, but in gel form, and comes in either 5g sachets or a pump dispenser. The sachets each contain 50mg of testosterone, which is about 10 times stronger than the daily dose of the AndroFeme 1. This means that you don't apply a full Testogel sachet every day – you use one sachet over the course of ten days or so. You could try applying one-tenth of a sachet every day, which might be messy and inaccurate, but many HRT specialists do suggest this method. One full sachet rubbed into your inner thigh every seven to ten days may also work – or half a tube every five days? – but some women may feel a bit too 'testosteroney' if they lash it all on at once. It's generally a case of trial and error. There are no clear rules about this, the main thing is to be cautious not to overuse it. Also, just to note that if you are using a full pump/sachet once every ten days and you go for your testosterone blood test, you could register a high level if you apply a full whack in the three to five days before the blood is taken – so skip or delay it that week.

Testogel also comes in a pump bottle, but the potency is slightly weaker than the gel so the dosage instructions are different (I know: *why make it easy?!*). The pump needs to be primed when you use it for the first time, so when you take off the cover, press the plunger pump down three times and throw away whatever comes out in the first of those three pumps. One full pump will give you 20mg of testosterone, so you will need two pumps (40mg), which ought to cover you for the next seven to ten days.

Testim

This is a similar product to Testogel, although I haven't seen it used recently. It used to come in tubes, and a single 50mg tube would deliver 50mg testosterone. So one tube over the course of seven to ten days is ideal.

Tostran

This is another brand of testosterone that your pharmacist might offer that is slightly stronger than Testogel or Testim. It is a 2 per cent gel that usually comes as a pump. It is more concentrated than Andro-Feme 1, but less concentrated than Testogel/Testim. Each single pump of Tostran delivers 10mg of testosterone. Women need to get an average of 50mg every seven to ten days, which is the goal, so you need to use about five pumps every week. One easy way to do this is to use one pump of Tostran every day, from Monday to Friday, but none on the weekend. I have also heard of clinics suggesting women use it every other day.

KEY TAKEAWAYS

☒ No blood test is needed to prescribe testosterone unless there is a suspicion you already have abnormally high levels of it. However, the most recent recommendations advise that we should measure your levels prior to use.

☒ If you are taking testosterone, you must have blood tests to monitor your testosterone levels one to three months after starting it, and yearly thereafter.

☒ If you do experience any side effects, they can usually be reversed by stopping the testosterone.

☒ As a woman, you must always apply testosterone directly on to the skin. Women never use testosterone tablets.

13. Local vaginal oestrogen – preserving and protecting the vagina

Local vaginal oestrogen is an option for managing menopause symptoms associated with changes in the vagina and pelvic area. Perhaps surprisingly, even when a person is on ample systemic oestrogen and progestagen hormone therapy, they often need local vaginal oestrogen as well. For thoroughness, therefore, I want to give local oestrogen the same treatment as the three sex hormones you get in HRT, seeing as it's often used in conjunction with HRT.

Take a look back at Chapter 4 (especially pages 40–44) for a recap of the symptoms known collectively as the genito-urinary syndrome of the menopause (GSM).

Benefits of local vaginal oestrogen therapy

Using local vaginal oestrogen products alone or in conjunction with systemic HRT oestrogen/progestagen will correct most, if not all, of the symptoms of GSM.

Using a good dose (i.e. as directed, depending on product) of vaginal oestrogen for the first two weeks of treatment usually makes an improvement in symptoms such as vaginal dryness, vaginal burning and irritation, and sexual symptoms such as lack of lubrication and painful, dry penetrative sex. Typically, the first two weeks that you are starting on vaginal oestrogen, you need to use loads of it. Thereafter, you pull back to a maintenance dose, which is much lower.

Vaginal oestrogen can also help with urinary symptoms, such as urgency (needing to race to the toilet to pee), frequency (peeing too often and at night), pain when passing urine, and recurrent urinary tract infections (UTIs).

At the risk of sounding repetitive: as these problems do not tend to improve with age, the answer is to keep using your vaginal oestrogen and don't plan to come off it – you may need to be buying and applying your vaginal oestrogen well past your pension age!

Non-dangerous side effects of local vaginal oestrogen therapy

These are the most common side effects.

- Oestrogen in the vagina can be linked to fungal infections. Some people are persecuted with thrush when they are on the contraceptive pill or pregnant, so it is not surprising that this can happen when they start taking local vaginal oestrogen.
- The cream or the pessary may sting you either outside, on your vulva, or inside your vagina when you first start using it. This is because there are often many little abrasions – you may not see them, but they are there – like tiny paper-cuts in an oestrogen-deprived vagina. As the oestrogen starts working optimally, the tissue will heal and thicken, but the first few days may cause more irritation than relief.
- Some people are sensitive to any and all creams and can get an allergic reaction to either the oestrogen itself or to the goop that the pessary/pellet/cream comes in. At first you may get heat, pain and/or itching from the oestrogen pessary, but this should settle. About 1 in 100 women experience vulvo-vaginal burning, itch, pain and stinging when they pee. Only about 1 in 1,000 women experience vaginal discharge and anorectal discomfort, so that's uncommon.

And finally, one thing being post-menopausal has going for it is that I have the cleanest knickers. It is hard to tell if they've even been worn because nothing is secreted from the vagina any more. However, if you use local vaginal oestrogen that will change, and you might be washing knickers for real again. (You can tell how much I hate laundry!)

Fixes for local vaginal oestrogen side effects

Obviously, using less until you get a nice balance may be necessary. If in doubt, stop it and try again with a lower dose, and if problems persist for more than a few weeks, discuss it with your prescribing doctor or nurse.

A note of caution regarding local vaginal oestrogen therapy

There are no risks that I know of clinically – or personally, or anecdotally – but you wouldn't be reassured reading the product information leaflet on some of these medicines. They often say things like:

- *Using oestrogen alone may increase your chance of getting cancer of the uterus (womb)*: well, perhaps, if you are putting it into your bloodstream, but *not* when you just use it in the vagina! This has never happened.
- *Using oestrogen alone may increase your chances of getting strokes or blood clots*: well, a little, if you swallow oestrogen tablets, but not when you just use it in your vagina.
- *Using oestrogens with progestins may increase your chances of getting heart attacks, strokes, breast cancer, or blood clots*: again, sure, a little, when you are putting it in your bloodstream, but not when you just put it in your vagina!

Do you sense a trend? It is as if the manufacturers just copied and pasted the warnings from a box of regular oestrogen for HRT.

Local vaginal oestrogen is safe for you to try. As I explained in Chapter 5 there is, however, an important concern when it comes to people on aromatase inhibitors (AIs) as part of breast cancer treatment. An abundance of caution is the rule of thumb with breast cancer, and that's fair enough. The British Menopause Society suggests that people with a breast cancer diagnosis should try non-hormonal vaginal moisturizers and/or lubricants first and, if they are not helpful, then try local vaginal oestrogens. People on AIs should probably speak to their oncologist about possibly getting off the AIs and maybe trying

Tamoxifen, which is usually kinder to the vagina. But this applies only if you are allowed to do so by your doctor – it's not always possible or permissible to swap cancer drugs around. (See Chapter 18, pages 216–17 for more on this.)

KEY TAKEAWAYS

☒ Local vaginal oestrogen is applied directly to the 'local' area, i.e. straight on to the vagina. This means it doesn't pass through your liver or blood in any significant way.

☒ You can use local vaginal oestrogen in conjunction with your HRT blend. It can deliver extra protection for your vagina.

☒ The primary purpose of local vaginal oestrogen is to protect you against the highly undesirable symptoms of GSM.

☒ The warnings on the leaflet in a box of local vaginal oestrogen are not always accurate. While regular HRT is almost always contraindicated after breast cancer, local vaginal oestrogen almost never is. Speak to your doctor or see the BMS/Women's Health Concern online information sheets on local vaginal oestrogen (www.womens-health-concern.org).

14. Bio-identical (aka body-identical) HRT explained

If you choose to go the HRT route to manage your perimenopausal or menopausal symptoms, that must be based on an in-depth discussion with your doctor that covers all aspects of your health and circumstances and identifies the best solution for you. Also, you need to be aware that your HRT needs might change over time. You might start off on one combination of hormones but find, for example, that you need more oestrogen as time goes by. Alternatively, as you get further from fifty years of age, you may need less oestrogen – you could even reduce the dose yourself (but you must *not* reduce the progestagen dose without talking to your prescriber). So, yearly HRT reviews are essential, even when you are on a good cocktail that you feel is working.

In Chapter 9 I explained how HRT got a bad image after the Women's Health Initiative (WHI) study, which linked HRT to an increased risk of breast cancer. Since then, some of the study authors have apologized for how their findings were communicated and interpreted, but it did cause a lot of damage. Apart from all its other flaws, the HRT used in the WHI study was the old stuff – an equine urine-based HRT that's rarely prescribed in Ireland. We've come a long way since then, modern science is working with a much greater level of knowledge, and the lab-produced HRT used nowadays is largely plant-based, so you aren't looking to horse pee for your health and well-being, I'm happy to say.

In this chapter I drill down into two approaches to HRT you may come across, and how they are created and regulated:

- bio-identical HRT, and
- compounded HRT.

This should give you the knowledge and confidence you need to understand what your GP, or other sources, might be recommending to you.

Before proceeding, I need to say something about terminology here. You'll see the words 'bio-identical' and 'body-identical' in relation to regulated and unregulated HRT, and I use them both here as well. Some people make a song and dance about these terms and how they should be used, but to be honest, whatever terms are used, the really important words for you to learn about in this chapter are **regulated** and **unregulated** – that's what you need to be aware of when making HRT choices. The fact is that 'bio-identical' and 'body-identical' are used interchangeably by most medical folks, so don't see them as meaning 'better than' or 'more natural' or anything like that – they are just handy labels when talking about these HRT products.

The safest option – regulated bio-identical HRT

A hormone is a chemical that helps regulate the activity of cells and tissues and other hormones in the body. 'Bio-identical' hormones are hormones that are chemically identical to the hormones made naturally in our body, therefore we *assume* they will have an effect on us that is 'identical' to the effect of our own natural hormones – and they usually do! That's a very simple explanation of the whole thing, but it's basically bio-engineered hormones that ought to behave in your body in the same way your original hormones behave.

Regulated bio-identical HRTs (rBHRT) are manufactured by pharmaceutical companies in their laboratories and contain chemicals that mimic the work of the natural hormones in the body – oestrogen and progestagen – but they are molecularly identical to the hormones produced by your ovaries. That's why it's called 'bio-identical' – in other words, these lab-created replacements perform in an identical manner to your natural biological hormones, thereby balancing and then replacing those fluctuating or reduced hormones in your body.

Hormones can be manufactured from plant or animal sources, or even synthesized, from scratch, in the lab. So, even though we expect bio-identical hormone products to have a 'natural' impact on our bodies, they are not necessarily sourced from nature as such. They might derive from a plant source, but the chemical in that source will need to be extracted from that source to create the bio-identical hormone, so it's sort of a mix of natural base and synthetic process.

Regulated bio-identical HRT is termed 'regulated' because it is licensed for sale in pharmacies. The HRT isn't made in your local pharmacy. It is manufactured in labs, but if classed as 'regulated', it means it has gone through all the necessary trials and ticked all the boxes to prove its safety and efficacy to the standard required for doctors to prescribe it, and for it to go on sale in pharmacies. So, when you get HRT with the word 'regulated' attached, you know it means that this product has been through a full testing programme before anyone is allowed to sell it to you.

Now, I can't give you specifics on the manufacturing processes involved because I've never been in such a lab, and the information available on the processes involved is limited (although take a look at the Notes and Sources of Further Information at the back of the book if you want to know more). It's a crazy, complicated chemical process – but this is also true in the human body! The whole thing is complex because our bodies are beautifully complicated. The chemical processes that are quietly happening inside you all day long are mind-blowing, really, when you get right down to it.

The fact that it's possible to create bio-identical hormones in a lab is a testament to how far we've come in terms of medical science and bio-engineering – and while most of us struggle to understand all the chemistry underpinning it, we can be grateful that science makes these hormones available to us for use in HRT products.

In terms of licensing those products for use by you and me, the medicines licensing authority in Ireland is called the Health Products Regulatory Authority (HPRA). It regulates medicines for use in humans and animals (veterinary products), and grants licences. Their website (www.hpra.ie) is useful, in fact, because you can search any product to see if it has a licence in Ireland – and licence number and other information is listed.

However, it's worth noting that not all good and reliable HRT products will be listed with the HPRA. A drug manufacturer needs to apply to the HPRA to be granted a licence specifically for Ireland and Irish patients, and the fees for this application process are high. If the company isn't going to make lots of money from sales of a specific drug, it may not be bothered to apply for a *specific* Irish licence. But if a well-known product recommended by the British Menopause Society (BMS) has licensing in other modern European countries, then Irish doctors might recommend that product to Irish patients. (This is called prescribing 'off-licence' – more on this below). So, for example, at this time no copper coils have a specific Irish licence, but we use them in Ireland all the time, have done for over fifty years, our rationale being that certain copper IUDs have a pan-European licence. Certainly, if something is licensed for use in the UK, doctors in Ireland usually would not hesitate to recommend it, with or without a specific Irish HPRA licence.

Bio-identical hormones licensed for use in Ireland

Progestagen

The only bio-identical progestagen available in Ireland is micronized progesterone (P4), sold under the brand name Utrogestan. It comes as a tablet that may be swallowed or inserted vaginally. However, if you read the manufacturer's instructions, nowhere does it mention its use as part of an HRT combination. So, here is a good example of a fabulous product being used to treat a condition without having a specific Irish licence for that purpose. I believe Utrogestan falls under the category of an 'exempt medicinal product' – meaning it is okay for a prescriber to use it for HRT in Ireland because it is approved for this purpose elsewhere in Europe.

Oestrogen

There are lots of bio-identical oestrogens available for HRT in Ireland – for example, 17-beta estradiol is available as patches sold under the brand names Evorel and Estradot. There is the oestrogen spray Lenzetto, and the gels called Divigel and Oestrogel. All but the spray are licensed in Ireland, but the spray has a UK licence, so we run with that.

What about off-label/off-licence use of standard pharmacy HRT?

When you buy a prescription HRT product in the pharmacy, it naturally comes with a full label describing the type of HRT and the recommended usage. The big instruction sheet inside — the one that folds out from tiny to map-like — is filled with important information on usage, side effects, et cetera. You're used to this from every product you buy in the pharmacy, so this is standard practice. But what happens if your doctor would like to deviate from the recommended standard practice described on the product?

The menopause societies warn prescribers like me to be very cautious about prescribing standard pharmacy HRT products in unconventional ways, because there may have been few trials or studies of the product being used in this way, at this dose or in this situation. Medicines are to be used 'as labelled' — that is, if it says *take 200mg three times a day*, it is because the clinical trials of that drug have shown it to be safe and effective at that dose. The trials are a big part of the long and expensive process of bringing a new drug to the market, and as doctors we try to respect the recommendations. Yet, there might be times when we bend the rules, for example, when we feel you could get by with a lower dosage, or perhaps start with a lower dosage and review the outcome.

This is not common practice, by the way, and it only occurs for certain medications. Where the goal of a medication is to stop a bad thing from happening — like, for example, your blood pressure medication that keeps your BP normal so you don't get a stroke or a heart attack — then we, and you, should *never* mess about with the dose. (I am talking to you, Mom!) But where the goal of the product is to just feel a little better — for example, when using pain medication — then possibly you can use less, if you don't need more. So, we do, at times, bend the rules — but usually only when we know that it is relatively safe to do so and when we suspect that there will likely never be a large clinical trial to look at the situation at hand. When we do that, we are prescribing 'off label'.

Prescribing medicines outside the labelled recommendations creates some extra work for us as doctors. The Irish Medical Council tells us that when we recommend a drug outside the labelled recommendation we need to do all of the following.

- Make darn sure there is a good reason to do it and that it is something that doctors with expertise in the relevant area recommend.
- Make sure the patient understands that using the product in this way is not part of the 'labelled' recommendations and *why* you want them to use the drug in this way.
- Explain thoroughly and exactly how this medicine is going to be used, and provide written or at least online instructions for the patient to refer to when they leave the surgery and forget what you told them to do. (The leaflet inside the pack will be giving conflicting information, so it's no good to you any more.)

Going off-label usually arises when a patient has a consultation with a specialist who has a broader knowledge of a disease and how to treat it than most doctors might have. A specialist might have been to clinical meetings where new therapies are presented, or new ways to use current therapies are being researched, and there they might learn that this drug really works but you need to use Y amount of it instead of the usual Z amount that is on the leaflet.

A great example of this is local vaginal oestrogen. We know that low-dose constant use of vaginal oestrogen will not be absorbed into the bloodstream in volumes strong enough to affect your womb or your breasts, and we often recommend it for women who would be better off avoiding systemic HRT – like after breast cancer diagnosis, for instance. However, the label on all local vaginal oestrogen products will say, *Do not use if you have been diagnosed with breast cancer.* So, when we recommend it for patients with a breast cancer diagnosis, we are going off-label, but we are doing so based on reliable knowledge.

I go to as many of the UK, European and international meetings on menopause that I can get to, and we often hear of new and interesting treatments that are being used in other clinics or in other countries, with good results. I'm open to all that's coming down the line, so back in my own clinic I might say to a patient, 'I heard about this, it isn't standard procedure yet, but they do it over there, and there's no reason to believe it might be dangerous. What do you think?' We look at it together and make a decision based on all of the available evidence – and sometimes that decision is to go off-label, do things differently and monitor closely.

In the case of local vaginal oestrogen, for example, I know the label recommends lowest dose for shortest period of time, but I also know that the BMS guidelines say that I can recommend as much as is required for as long as the patient likes. I know this is backed up by clinical trials, so I can trust the guidelines on this. As a result, when I recommend vaginal oestrogen to my patients, once there are no *genuine* contraindications of any kind, I tell them they can stay on it for as long as they like, if it's helping them.

Another common example of off-label prescribing is when we offer testosterone as part of HRT. Testosterone gel for perimenopausal patients has only one licensed (labelled) reason for use and that is low sex drive. We use it all the time for exactly that purpose. But I suspect – and other colleagues agree from listening to our patients and reading about the experiences of other menopause specialists throughout the world – that testosterone therapy can help with a few other menopause symptoms as well, such as poor cognitive ability and low energy. For this reason, we sometimes recommend testosterone as part of HRT for women who have other symptoms besides low sex drive. The same goes for using the men's male hormone gels in menopausal women, as the labelled instructions for these products all say, *For use in men* – apart from the Australian AndroFeme 1, which is specifically labelled for use in women.

There isn't a problem with going off-label once you, the patient, understand that's what it is and why we are recommending it. If you're being recommended an 'off-label' product by your doctor, just ensure that you receive a written or online explanation as to how to use it and why it's being prescribed in this manner for you.

A more experimental approach (and not one most menopause experts favour) – 'compounded' bio-identical HRT

There is growing awareness about 'compounded HRT', which refers to menopause hormone products that are usually made up in small, private laboratories. They blend together different types of HRT hormones in creams and lozenges. I do not know where they get the raw materials from to create the products but they claim to be able to blend them in all different combinations and dosages, to 'suit your individual need'.

I can give you a little bit of the history here, just to show how this practice was born and developed. Most of the 'compounding' business started in the USA, where the only form of HRT they had in the pharmacy for many decades was horse urine oestrogen plus the progestagen MPA. Women there did not want that stuff – and they *really* did not want it after the WHI results were published in 2002 showing that small (but heavily hyped) increase in breast cancer rates. In response, medical entrepreneurs there looked to Europe and saw how we had lots of other types of HRT available, many of which were identical to human female oestrogen and progestagen. That was a great alternative, right there. But rather than try and get the FDA to approve European products, they decided to mix some up themselves – and the private compounded HRT cocktail was born. These private prescribers made a virtue of being outside the mainstream of FDA-approved HRT options by presenting their products as more bespoke and specialized and away from the sinister grip of 'Big Pharma'. The claim that compounded HRT is 'tailor-made' and 'natural' has created an impression that it is perhaps safer/better/smarter than standard HRT. There was an element of playing into patients' understandable need to feel that they were getting something very responsive to their individual needs. I cannot emphasize enough that a well-informed GP who has an interest in this area of medicine will be able to give you a genuinely bespoke service, and all using very well-researched products.

A private lab will create a bottle of cream for you or give you a 28-pack of little sugar squares that may claim to have xmcg of estriol plus *x*mcg of estradiol plus *x*mcg of progesterone plus *x*mcg of DHEA testosterone in a single squirt of cream or a single lozenge. To reiterate: these costly products are not subject to the same scrutiny as standard body-identical HRT from a pharmacy. Pharma companies are legally required to put an accurate list of all the constituents of any medicinal product on the leaflet, compounding labs are not. Secret shopper reports conducted in the USA, where the compounded products have been tested in accredited labs, were found to have nowhere near the amount of hormone in the bottle or pack as was claimed by the label. The excipients (cream/thickeners/preservatives) were also found to be inaccurately represented – which could be a big problem, say if you were allergic to something.

You can't buy compounded products in the pharmacy, so most people source them online and there are some doctors in Ireland recommending or even selling them. However, conventional menopause doctors do not always like or support compounded HRT, so there can be a conflict between the doctor's and the patient's perceptions of it. Let's look at the pros and cons.

The BMS doesn't recommend using hormone products from private laboratories, for several reasons.

- Regulated pharmaceutical laboratories are supposed to be monitored by outside authorities for purity, potency and safety of the drugs they manufacture. Private compounded labs are not subject to this oversight. This is why these products are often described as 'natural' – that word may actually denote that a product is unlicensed for pharmaceutical use. This is the main objection to compounded HRT: that products can slip through the net of clinical trials. Doctors generally shy away from using pharmaceuticals that have not had decent clinical studies carried out on them for dose, safety, purity, side effects, et cetera. Every country has a medicines regulatory authority that checks out medicines and products to keep us as safe as possible from products and drugs that may do more harm than good. Privately compounded HRT products do not need to be approved by the usual authorities because they are not going to be offered for sale through the pharmacies.

- Compounded HRT products may often mix different oestrogens together – a little estrone (E1) and some estradiol (E2) and a little estriol (E3) for good measure – even though we have no way of knowing what effect the blend of these different oestrogens might have on oestrogen-sensitive tissues in the body, especially those in the breast.
- Privately compounded HRT drugs may have micronized progesterone* in a cream that you are meant to apply every day, even though we know that absorbing progesterone through the skin, especially the gentle micronized progesterone, is unpredictable. I know of no menopause/HRT expert group that supports the use of transdermal progesterone. We know that too little progesterone in the blood may not adequately protect your womb-lining from the oestrogen you are also taking and can leave it at risk of cancer. You will never see micronized progesterone in a pharmaceutical/regulated patch or cream because no studies support the use of progesterone through the skin,† based on the fact that you may not absorb enough to safeguard your womb-lining. That might change in the future, but for now it is a no-no.

The problem is that while there is HRT hormone in these products – no question about it – they are not regulated and very little information is forthcoming on the processes involved, therefore it can be unclear how much is included or under what exact conditions the products were made. One of the reasons it has taken years to address the upswing in HRT demand is that licensed manufacturers can't just create a new batch of HRT to meet demand – it takes months or years

---

* A quick reminder: progesterone is the hormone released by the ovaries that's important for the menstrual cycle and pregnancy because it changes the cells of the womb-lining to prepare it for a fertilized egg to take up residence.
† We do have access to an approved progesterone product for skin use in the UK and Ireland – it is called norethisterone acetate (NET) and is found in the patch Evorel Conti and similar products. But NET is a stronger, artificial progestagen with *proven* reliable absorbability through the skin. Otherwise, micronized progesterone in tablet form (Utrogestan) is the product we favour in HRT.

to set up a new factory and get industry-standard approval. But that doesn't apply to the private labs.

Lastly – and this is my own personal objection to bespoke, compounded HRT – it is really expensive. Now, HRT is already pricey enough at about €12–€20 per month for the simple tablet options. If you go for the, arguably better, bio-identical HRT, that is even more costly, going up to about €20–€30 a month,* and there's extra on that again if you want to add in the testosterone. If you opt for a Mirena coil (see next chapter), that can run into hundreds of euro. In an ideal world it should be free to all, but we are a long way off that in Ireland, so for now we try to be aware of end-user costs and to work with our patients to find affordable solutions. On that score, the compounded preparations can be wickedly expensive and yet are in no way superior to standard bio-identical HRT out of the local pharmacy. I have had patients spending €80–€100 each month on these creams and lozenges, and that is on top of the couple of hundred euro they spent to get the advice and the prescription. It's a lot of money.

So why is compounded HRT becoming more popular, then? Well, that brings us to the cons. The not-so-surprising thing about compounded HRT products is that they are often highly effective, and the people who can afford to use them usually love them and shout their love from the rooftops. This efficacy is mainly because they often contain pretty high doses of oestrogen. In terms of regulated HRT, although we will go as high as we need to in order to control your symptoms, we don't want to throw the kitchen sink at you from the get-go, so we usually start you off with a modest dose to see if that gets the job done and then slowly increase the dose until we find the *lowest effective amount* you need to be well.

Another reason I think so many patients want to try compounded HRT products is that you see adverts for them online all the time, and since it can be hard to get a good menopause consultation from your GP – they may not have the right level of expertise (though this is improving all the time, except that now there is a shortage of GPs

---

* My editor tells me she's paying nearly €40 a month for patches at her local pharmacy (in Dublin city centre). I've told her that sounds pricey, and she needs to shop around!

and they are run off their feet!) – you would be forgiven for turning to an online clinic that promised you results. It can be so demoralizing when you are struggling, you are sure you know what is wrong and what you need, but the local doctor doesn't get seem to get you. Some of the more expensive private menopause services, on the other hand, are sometimes readily available and seem to have all the time in the world. Some of the really expensive ones can be particularly appealing because they may suggest that you can get your hormone levels measured via blood or saliva testing, with the promise that this will allow them to calculate the exact amount of hormone you will require in your bespoke HRT. These tests are not a standard part of any menopause specialist consultation because there is no scientifically accepted way to identify hormone levels via saliva testing – sex hormones by their nature fluctuate, and no saliva test can accurately identify hormone levels – and we only do blood hormone levels when we suspect early/premature menopause. For most patients over the age of forty-five, bloods are almost never necessary.

Also, be aware that if you do an online menopause consultation with a private doctor outside of Ireland, they cannot prescribe Irish pharmacy HRT for you. It requires a prescription from an Irish-registered doctor with an Irish Medical Council registration number to get medicine from a pharmacy in Ireland. That means you might need to get a GP to rewrite the script for you, and most doctors in Ireland will not agree to do this unless they have their own expertise in this area. Of course, if the private menopause doctor prescribes a privately compounded product, you can buy that directly from them and skip the pharmacy altogether – easy-peasy – except you are now a few hundred euro poorer and you don't have all the regulatory checks and balances to rely on in your unlicensed HRT product.

What you have to be wary of is falling into a trap of believing that compounded products, advertised as 'bio-identical' or 'natural', are safer or better for you. There is no evidence at all to suggest that compounded HRT products are more natural and safer than standard, body-identical, prescription HRT. The term 'bio-identical' does not mean tailor-made or extra-special. Any doctor in Ireland can prescribe bio-identical or body-identical HRT through the pharmacy using regulated, tested pharmaceutical products. Moreover, you can get bio-identical HRT on the GMS (medical card) and Drugs Payment schemes, so there is no need to be paying through the nose to get your HRT through a private compounding service.

KEY TAKEAWAYS

- Bio-identical regulated HRT is readily available from the pharmacies in Ireland and usually covered by the Medical Card or DP schemes.

- Compounded HRT is not 'better' or 'safer' than regulated HRT. This claim I think arose out of the USA where it was hard to buy anything other than horse urine HRT tablets for many decades. I am a prescriber and a user of HRT and I would never use an HRT product from a private lab.

- Not all medicines are licensed for the way we use them in Ireland, but if there are good guidelines around this unlicensed use and your doctor knows what they are doing, then you are okay to use them.

- The rule of thumb with HRT is to use the *lowest effective dose*, with *effective* being the operative word. So, if someone feels 99 per cent better on a 50mcg patch, I would not recommend going up to 75mcg just to see if that last 1 per cent can be corrected – unless she is unhappy, and then we can talk. Always start low-ish, usually with 50mcg of oestrogen, and then go up if need be. (The exception to this might be POI sufferers, who often need more oestrogen.)

- Another good reason not to start too high with oestrogen doses is that high, sustained doses of oestrogen are more likely to precipitate side effects like headache and nausea, but if we start slow and low, those side effects are less likely. Bear this in mind when discussing options with your GP.

15. HRT and unscheduled bleeding

Unscheduled or unexpected bleeding refers to any bleeding from the vagina that was not anticipated – either as part of your natural, monthly period bleed or the timed bleeds that you can get from hormone medications such as the combined pill or HRT. It is very common for this to happen when you are on HRT, especially when you first try it. Of course, unscheduled bleeding (UB) is always a nuisance, but the worst part is that it can be extremely unsettling and upsetting and might cause some people to panic and come off their HRT needlessly. And as well as causing needless worry for the patient, it can also cause anxiety in your GP, who may rush you into the gynaecology services for an unnecessary referral.

The reason we worry so much about unscheduled bleeding is that all doctors know UB, especially if it occurs after we thought your last period had come and gone forever, can be a sign of womb-lining cancer. If a lady is *not* on HRT and is older (over the age of fifty-five) and has completely finished her periods, they should never start up again. If they do, that could be the first red flag for womb-lining cancer. The problem is that HRT, by its very nature, rejuvenates the dry womb-lining and can make you bleed. So there can be a lot of confusion – is this just an unexpected/unscheduled bleed from your HRT hormones or is it something more sinister?

Unexpected bleeding on HRT can manifest in different ways. You may not have had a natural period for many years, only to bleed suddenly again, out of the blue, soon after starting your HRT. Or you may already be experiencing a period-type bleed but now find that you are bleeding in between expected periods, at a time when an expected bleed is not due. This unscheduled bleeding may be heavy and there may even be 'flooding', which is when you bleed so much, it leaks out on to your clothes or bedsheets – a flow so heavy that a pad or tampon can't contain it. It may be prolonged and persistent, with no real pattern.

The bad news and the good news is that it is extremely common among HRT users. Up to 80 per cent of women will get unscheduled bleeding or light spotting in the first six months of taking an HRT product. Hopefully this high occurrence indicates that there's no need for panic, no need to race straight into the gynae clinic, although the bleeding does need to be reported and monitored by the doctor who prescribed your HRT. If you are on a *sequential/cyclical* HRT product – one that is supposed to make you get periods – you have an 80 per cent chance of experiencing UB in the first few months of starting your HRT, but by nine months this should have reduced to as little as 10 per cent.

In Chapter 9, I described cyclical and continuous HRT – cyclical means you still get a period, while continuous means you shouldn't, in theory, get any more periods. This comes down to how you use progestagen – either daily or on/off. The BMS guidelines suggest that:

- if you're under 50 and have had a natural period in the last 18–24 months, then you should take cyclical HRT – and you'll still get a period;
- if you have had no bleeding for 18–24 months, you can take continuous progestagen and you shouldn't get any bleeding at all (eventually);
- if you're over 50 and have not had a period for 12 months, you can take continuous progestagen and you shouldn't get any bleeding at all (eventually).

All this comes with the warning that on both types of HRT – cyclical or continuous – you can experience bleeding at unexpected times, usually when you first start your HRT, while your womb-lining gets used to the hormone. More than half of patients taking progestagen in the '2 weeks on/2 weeks off' regime can bleed before day 11 of the progestagen-taking days of the month. For continuous progestagen users, if you are on a 'no more periods' type of HRT, you can still get UB, even if it has been many months or years since your last period. The possibility should be lower for you, but it can still occur.

One of the main reasons why we have rules for deciding who gets a 'no period' HRT cocktail, and which patients will continue to accept the possibility of a period, is to minimize the risk of U B and avoid unnecessary worry, tests and referrals to hospital. I occasionally have met patients who need and want HRT, but who ask for 'the kind that turns your periods off'. I wish there was such a thing! But I have to tell you, no such HRT product exists. I might be able to lighten your bleed with a Mirena coil, but if your ovaries are still punching out some sex hormone, you *will* bleed and I can't stop that. Best I can do is put some manners on it.

Now, having said that it's very common, please do not ignore U B : if you experience it, you should report it to your doctor, and it should be monitored. If it sounds innocent and likely to have resulted from your HRT, there are some established fixes we can try (described further down). For many people those will sort it out. If needs be, we can get an ultrasound scan and maybe refer you to a gynae specialist, but we only need to do this if the bleeding has not responded to one of the well-known fixes within six months, or if it is causing you so much concern and inconvenience that you simply cannot tolerate it.

It's also the case that you might get referred to a gynae straight away if you are in a 'high-risk group' for cancer of the womb-lining, such as being very obese, have Lynch syndrome in the family (see Chapter 7), are a very heavy smoker, or if you have been on Tamoxifen recently. But even if this does apply to you, you can continue to try new combinations products, in consultation with your doctor, while awaiting the appointment.

Why do some women who start HRT bleed more than others?

When it comes to periods there are many factors that influence when we bleed, how long for and the amount of blood we lose. This will bring you right back to Leaving Cert biology, but just to recap, here's a breakdown of your average menstrual cycle.

- Days 1–7: menstruation/bleeding – duration varies.
- Days 8–12: follicular/proliferative phase – womb-lining builds up again after the period.

- Days 13–15: ovulation – release of egg from the ovary, flows down the fallopian tube.
- Days 16–28: luteal/secretory phase – womb-lining continues to thicken and egg is either fertilized, which means pregnancy might occur, or egg isn't fertilized and menstruation occurs again.

Normally, during a typical, healthy menstrual cycle, four main hormones are responsible for all the phases of the cycle, and you've already made their acquaintance in the earlier chapters: FSH (follicle stimulating hormone), LH (luteinizing hormone), estradiol (E2) and progesterone (P4).

FSH levels rise from about day 1 or 2 of the beginning of a menstrual cycle, i.e. the start of a period. FSH prompts the maturing follicles in the ovary to prepare for that month's egg release. Those follicles will compete to appoint a dominant follicle, which is usually the follicle with the most FSH receptors on it. In response to rising FSH, oestrogen levels slowly start to rise as well. The increasing oestrogen level in turn slows down womb-lining shedding and 'turns off' the period after about the fifth day of your cycle. It does this through a complex interaction with oestrogen receptors in the womb-lining.

After the period stops, steady levels of oestrogen keep coming from the ovary and this causes a thickening in the lining of the womb, which we will need if we are going to support and nurture a pregnancy. The textbooks call this the 'proliferative phase' of the uterine cycle; I call it the 'stuff is getting chunky' phase.

Under the influence of the brain's luteinizing hormone (LH), a dominant follicle (or two!) will rupture and release its egg (ovulation), which then flows down the fallopian tube. The now empty follicle shrivels into a collection of hormone-producing cells – it is yellow in colour and, weirdly, it looks to me like a lemon slice when I can find it during an ultrasound. It is called the *corpus luteum*, which is Latin for yellow body (maybe they didn't know the Latin for lemon slice!). It produces increasing amounts of progesterone in the hopes that fertilization will occur up in the tube and that, sometime in the next five days or so, a fertilized egg will arrive down into a womb with a plump juicy lining, ready to accept that egg into its tissue (implantation).

If a fertilized egg does not get implanted in the womb-lining, the empty follicle (yellow body) eventually gives up producing progesterone. The fall in progesterone lets the now-thickened womb-lining start to peel away and be released from the walls of the womb (menstruation). You get a period, and we start all over again.

Now, perimenopausal and menopausal women have hormones coming at the womb-lining from all over the place. Perimenopausal women, in particular, still have significant amounts of oestrogen and progestagen in their blood anyway. So, what happens when you add HRT oestrogen and progestagen into that mix? When the oestrogen in HRT is introduced into the body, it can have an impact on the lining of the womb similar to the natural oestrogen in a menstrual cycle. The size of the endometrial vessels can increase in the presence of additional oestrogen. The thickness of the womb-lining will also increase in the presence of oestrogen. In other words, it prompts proliferation, or thickening of the womb-lining.

Progestagen, on the other hand, counteracts the proliferative impact of the oestrogen in HRT. It is the key hormone in preventing endometrial build-up, so the dose of progestagen needs to be high enough to reduce the volume of tissue build-up in the womb-lining. It is a finely balanced equilibrium – using enough oestrogen to control your symptoms, but then matching that with enough of the right progestagen to minimize womb-lining build-up and thus prevent UB.

There are lots of individual user response variations to different progestagens, oestrogens and their doses. Some progestagens are 'better' than others at preventing womb-lining build-up. One of the most popular progestagens we prescribe in Ireland, the bio-identical Utrogestan (discussed in the previous chapter), is less effective at womb-lining and bleed control. On the other hand, synthetic progestagens, particularly LNG, DSG and MPA, when given in low doses, can help reduce UB on HRT. Synthetic progestagens are not bio-identical and we sometimes recommend them intentionally as we know they are more likely to suppress the growth of your womb-lining and keep your periods light – or keep you bleed-free in some cases.

So, this tells you why you can experience UB when you start taking HRT – because the oestrogen in the HRT mimics natural oestrogen in the body and causes a 'period', of sorts. If the bleeding is not too heavy or disruptive, a watch-and-wait approach can be taken, with the hope that it will settle down in time as your body adjusts. Getting a balance between your own body's hormones and your HRT hormones may take some time. If you want to try and get rid of UB faster, the HRT cocktail can be tweaked to see if the bleeding will respond, although there is a very good chance of it resolving on its own if you can grin and bear it for a few months.

By the way, not taking the HRT correctly can cause UB: when your progestagen is prescribed as a separate entity to your oestrogen, *you have to take it!* If a patient neglects to take their progestagen as prescribed, they can get UB as a result. This is because every time you miss a progestagen tablet, it's like you are telling your womb-lining that you want to bleed.

Ruling out other causes of unscheduled bleeding

While there is an excellent chance that the HRT is the source of UB, it is not always the case. If we try lots of bleed-reducing options and combos with HRT, and we don't seem to be getting to the bottom of things, we will start looking for other explanations. We do this because there could be other causes of UB at work.

Some women get unexpected or heavy bleeding from *medical conditions*.

- The lining of the womb and how much it bleeds might be affected by structural things like fibroids and polyps. We will do an ultrasound scan or an MRI to try to rule out polyps, fibroids, ovarian cysts or cancers.
- Disorders like haemophilia or vaginal wall dryness or thyroid disease, as well as endometrial diseases like adenomyosis or endometrial cancers, can all cause UB, even in patients who are not taking HRT.

We may need to refer you to a gynae service to do blood tests and/or have a look directly at your womb-lining with a camera

(hysteroscopy – explained below) or directly at your pelvic structures via keyhole surgery or laparoscopy.

Drug interactions may contribute to UB on HRT. If you are on
other medicines that affect the way the liver processes drugs, or if you
are using oral HRT and you have a bowel absorption issue, you may
get UB on HRT because you might not be getting adequate levels
of the progestagen in your blood to control womb-lining bleeding.

Overweight women may be more likely to get UB on HRT. There
can be more of your own oestrogen – mostly E1, estrone – in your
blood if you are obese, so you may need more progestagen or a better
progestagen delivery route. The Mirena coil is often a good fix here
(see page 158).

Sexually transmitted infections (STIs) may cause UB on HRT. These
include infections like chlamydia or gonorrhoea. While STIs may
be more associated with younger people, obviously anyone who is
having sex can be exposed to a STI, so this should be investigated
and ruled out as well.

Cervical cancer may cause UB. Anyone who does not respond to
one or other of the 'hormonal fixes' needs to be examined, and that
includes having a look at your cervix. Smear tests do not detect cervical cancer – they are only useful in identifying pre-cancerous cell
changes. You need someone who knows what a cervix cancer looks
like to eyeball your cervix as part of a complete gynae review.

Possible fixes for unscheduled bleeding

There are a number of things we can recommend to tackle UB on
HRT. The options will be based on the type of HRT you are taking –
sequential or continuous.

Treatment options for patients on sequential HRT

Either *increase the dose* or *change the type of progestagen*. The commonly
prescribed bio-identical progesterone Utrogestan is notoriously gentle,
with a short half-life, that is to say it wears off pretty quickly. Synthetic
progestagens (progestins) – for example, Provera, Duphaston – may

be better for bleed control. Even better, a dose of a progestin called levonorgestrel (LNG) right in the endometrium is the best way to shut down undesired womb bleeding, so a Mirena coil might do the trick (see below).

Change the progestagen schedule. There are various dosage and timing combos your GP can suggest that may do the trick (for example, 200mg Utrogestan taken 2 weeks on/2 weeks off may be replaced by 300mg Utrogestan or 100mg Utrogestan taken 3 weeks on/1 week off).

Reduce the dose of oestrogen. This may reduce heavy/prolonged bleeding, but strangely enough it increases the possibility of spotting in the days leading up to the scheduled period days.

As a last resort, *stop the HRT.* Some people will do this themselves, out of fear or desperation. Abrupt discontinuation of HRT can lead to rebound vasomotor symptoms (hot flushes, night sweats, et cetera) which can be worse than the original menopause symptoms, as well as a return of other symptoms, like low mood and fatigue. When you come off any medical treatment very quickly, your symptoms can shoot back up just as quickly, and we call that 'rebounding'. In HRT terms, if you come off oestrogen slowly, you are less likely to get a return of your flushes and sweats, whereas if you stop overnight, you will get those symptoms back. For this reason, stopping HRT should be considered a 'when all else fails' strategy by both the doctor and the patient, but that is ultimately your decision.

Treatment options for patients on continuous HRT

There is a very common scenario whereby a non-bleeding patient starts on the Evorel Conti patch and then experiences bleeding. I recommend ignoring it for the first two to three months. If it's not gone by then, we need to change your HRT and maybe start to investigate at that point.

Add extra progestagen. One option is to leave you on the Evorel Conti patch but to add some extra progestagen in the form of oral norethisterone (NET), which is the same progestagen that is in the Evorel Conti patches. Another option would be to switch to Evorel (plain oestrogen) and use 200mg of Utrogestan instead of the NET in the Evorel Conti.

Use a Mirena coil. If the bleeding is wicked heavy and you are up for it, a Mirena coil might be the quickest and best solution. The intra-uterine contraceptive device (IUCD) we call Mirena is one of the best things to emerge in reproductive health care since the invention of the contraceptive pill. The Mirena prototype was developed in the 1970s. It works in a number of ways, but chiefly because it releases a continuous low dose of the progestin levonorgestrel (LNG), which prevents conception. The Mirena took ages to come to market and was finally launched by Bayer health in 1990. We didn't get going with the Mirena in Ireland until about 1998/99, but ever since that time it has become the backbone of GP and hospital gynaecology – with so many uses beyond its original purpose of contraception.

LNG is a strong progestin that helps keep the tissues of the womb-lining thin and stable. We use Mirena for so many medical things. It has been shown to be effective in preventing, slowing or treating:

- heavy periods (I have heard many gynaecologists say that they rarely have to consider doing hysterectomy for bleeding problems any more, because Mirena has changed the landscape of gynaecology)
- endometriosis /adenomyosis (endometriosis in your womb muscles)
- pelvic pain
- womb-lining hyperplasia (thickening)
- womb-lining polyps
- low-grade endometrial carcinoma or womb-lining carcinoma (slowing development)
- ovarian cancer (it is even suggested that wearing a Mirena may be protective).

As you can imagine, GPs and gynaes love the Mirena, and they can be a lifesaver for many patients on HRT. The Mirena releases 20mcg of LNG every 24 hours, which is enough progestagen to provide contraception for at least six years and enough progestagen to protect the womb-lining from HRT oestrogen for five years. The fun thing about Mirena is that it doesn't matter whether you have recently had periods or not, because it is suitable for everyone who wants one. So, a woman with a Mirena that has been in place for less than five years only needs oestrogen for HRT – and maybe some testosterone. The Mirena is fully taking care of her progestagen needs.

Once the Mirena has been in place for five years, you can either get a new Mirena or leave the old one there. You might choose to do this if, for example, you are using it to help with a gynaecological condition, such as heavy bleeding. If that's the case and it's staying put, you add in some oral or patch progestagen to your oestrogen HRT cocktail after the Mirena has been in for over five years. When it comes to treating UB in women on HRT, Mirena is a seriously good option.

When the usual fixes for UB don't work, then what?

If none of the fixes seems to be working and/or UB is alarming or heavy, then you'll be referred for in-depth investigations while your hormone doses and delivery routes are adjusted. The first step in an investigation is a detailed medical history review, to look for other clues. We will want to get an idea of the volume of blood loss and the functional disability caused. You don't absolutely need a vaginal examination straight away when UB on HRT first starts, but if it has been going on for weeks or months we will always do this. We might do it sooner if there is a suspicion of large fibroids or cervical disease.

The best next step is to get a scan, which is recommended in all cases of non-responsive UB on HRT. Even though we know the likelihood of serious disease is very low, we might pick up a fibroid or a cyst that can be treated and improve your quality of life on HRT.

There are a few different investigative options we can use.

Transvaginal ultrasound scan (TVUS)

This is a safe and cost-effective initial investigative test for UB, whether you are on HRT or not. It allows us to view the endometrium as well as other pelvic structures and areas, so as to rule out a variety of possible causes of UB. 'Transvaginal' means via the vagina, which means they need to put the probe into the lower end of your vagina. However, some patients don't want or cannot tolerate the probe being inserted into their vagina due to dryness/atrophy. If these conditions might cause you pain on a TVUS scan, one option is to ask the doctor to recommend some vaginal oestrogen and use it for two weeks before the internal scan (and then stay on it for as long as you want, if you like it!). If you feel the transvaginal scan really won't be possible, tell the doctor and the sonographer. Transabdominal scans are not always helpful for picking up abnormalities in the womb and pelvis, and you might be better off going straight to CT/MRI scan.

CT/MRI scan

If the sonographer identifies a disease or abnormality, they may recommend additional imaging, such as MRI or CT. These might be useful if other pelvic diseases are suspected, such as fibroids, polyps, cysts. If possible, people on sequential HRT should get their scan done in the first seven days off the progestagen. Even women on sequential HRT should have an endometrial thickness of less than 5mm if they get a scan at this stage of the month.

Following a healthy scan showing an endometrial thickness of less than 5 mm, the risk of endometrial cancer in post-menopausal women (which is less than 10 per cent anyway) decreases by a further 90 per cent for people both on and not on HRT. So, if you have UB on HRT but you are found to have a thin womb-lining, you're probably fine and you can continue to explore HRT options to shut down that bleeding.

Blind pipelle endometrial sampling

This involves gently sliding a pipelle tube – which is like a sucky straw – into your womb and collecting some of the tissue in there. The pipelle tube slides into the depth of your womb and sucks down any loose womb-lining tissue in there. It is easy to do in the GP or gynae office and quite painless, but it's done 'blind', without looking at the womb-lining tissues, so it's not entirely accurate. It may miss a small area of abnormality and should really only be offered while awaiting scan/hysteroscopy as it can miss up to 20 per cent of lesions, like polyps. A few GPs have the facility to do these samples in their surgery, but most will need to send you to the gynae outpatients for a pipelle sample.

Hysteroscopy

Hysteroscopy-directed endometrial sampling is the gold standard for uterine cavity evaluation. This is when a small probe with a camera on it is inserted through your vagina into your cervix and womb and allows us to see the inside of your womb – and you can watch it on a TV monitor if you like. From a doctor's point of view, this is the most effective investigation, but it does have some downsides. Obviously, it is invasive, and it can be painful and costlier than a scan or an office pipelle sample. The waiting list in some areas is quite long too, so all this needs to be factored in.

Hysteroscopic review is not usually necessary for people with UB on HRT who are low risk for serious disease. There is also the possibility that you may not be able to tolerate a scope test while you are awake, and you might be better off having this done asleep in the operating theatre – ask about this option if you have struggled to tolerate vaginal exams in the past. (If you have given birth, scope exams are usually quite tolerable.) Rarely, hysteroscopy can cause post-procedural infection and/or pain and also, very rarely, serious complications can occur (for example, uterine perforation, spread of malignant cells outside of the cavity), but these are very uncommon when done by an experienced provider.

It's good to know that a Mirena coil can be placed at the time of a hysteroscopy, but only if your GP thinks to prescribe one – and you remember to bring it with you! Ask your GP about this before your scope appointment because hospitals do not keep a stock of Mirena coils in the press.

D&C – with or without ablation and Mirena

A dilation and curettage (D&C) is performed under general anaesthetic (you'll be glad to hear) and involves stretching open the doorway to your womb (dilation) and scraping out the contents (curettage). You can also have an endometrial ablation for ongoing bleed problems. This takes place under the general anaesthetic as well. A laser-emitting probe is rolled around the womb-lining to cauterize it and prevent further bleeding. You can opt for a Mirena to be placed at the same time. If you have had an ablation but no Mirena was placed, your HRT must still contain progestagen as there may be some bits of endometrium left behind.

Hysterectomy

When absolutely all else fails, or when you love your HRT but you are fed up with the unresponsive UB, the womb can be removed. This is a big decision for any woman, and for her doctor, and must be considered carefully.

The pros of hysterectomy include the following.

- It is the ultimate fix if you are having womb problems, such as heavy/painful bleeds or pain/pressure from fibroids, womb cancer, et cetera.
- It is also the ultimate in contraception – not that we would ever do it just for that.
- It can be a great advantage if your periods are painful and you have tried everything else and you are fed up and want this rubbish over with.
- Many women report feeling great after hysterectomy.

These should be weighed against the cons of hysterectomy.

- It is a major surgery and you can develop complications.
- It involves a general anaesthetic and that brings risk.
- You can't drive for weeks afterwards.
- You are no longer able to have a baby.
- Some women regret having had a hysterectomy.

If both of your ovaries are removed, you'll definitely go straight into menopause. If one ovary is removed, you will still sometimes go straight into menopause!

Even when they leave the ovaries, menopause symptoms can kick off soon after your operation, although we're not sure why this happens. Perhaps the surgical disruption to the pelvis or its blood vessels is involved? We do not know. But do not let them tell you that leaving one or both ovaries will prevent menopause symptoms because the data do not bear that out!

There are studies to suggest that when a young woman has a hysterectomy but the ovaries are left behind, she is more at risk of depression. Is this a direct hormone consequence, or is it because you feel the loss of your fertility? We don't know.

UB and special cases

People on Tamoxifen therapy

Tamoxifen is associated with endometrial development and an increased risk of endometrial cancer. People currently on Tamoxifen will almost always have a thickened endometrium, so interpretation is difficult and therefore referral to a hysteroscopy service is recommended.

People on unopposed oestrogen

Unopposed oestrogen means using oestrogen on its own, without the addition of progestagen to balance the effects of the oestrogen. If you are on oestrogen and you have a womb, you *must* be on progestagen (or wearing a Mirena that is less than five years in). Using oestrogen on its own (unopposed) can put you at risk of developing womb-lining cell changes that could lead to cancer.

How could it happen that a woman would take unopposed oestrogen when it's not recommended? Sometimes I meet patients who have been recommended both oestrogen and progestagen but they decide not to take the progestagen because they don't like how it makes them feel. That is partly our fault for not impressing upon you the importance of taking your progestagen, whether you like it or not! It's also possible a doctor could prescribe oestrogen and forget to add the progestagen, maybe thinking your Mirena was in for less than five years.

People on compounded HRT

I went into detail about compounded HRT in the previous chapter. This covers the creams, lozenges and vaginal preparations sold online from 'specialist pharmacies' and these do not adhere to the same safeguards as regulated HRT. As a result, these products may not be adequately evaluated or controlled for either effectiveness or safety, which is why their use is not recommended by the BMS – but many women are on them. One of the biggest issues with compounded HRT cocktails is the habit of delivering progesterone via the skin – you get variable absorption when you use progesterone this way, and it may not provide adequate endometrial protection. If you have been on compounded HRT, talk to a menopause specialist and consider changing to regulated bio-identical HRT.

KEY TAKEAWAYS

- Unscheduled bleeding is very common when you start HRT. It is almost never a sign of disease and can usually be sorted by just waiting a while or changing the amount and/or type of your HRT hormones.
- If UB is not responding to HRT adjustments, it is time to get it investigated.
- If you are using oestrogen but *not* also getting some progestagen into your womb, you are at risk: don't do that.
- There are many gynaecological conditions that can also cause UB, and there are fixes for all of them.

16. HRT and your contraception choices

After reading all the stuff about the vagina and how age affects it, you'd be forgiven for swearing off sex forever! But that is NOT the message I am trying to send. This whole book is about optimism and empowerment and choice. Early menopause and POI can happen when you are very young. Perimenopause happens while you're still fairly young. And when it comes to post-menopausal women, I would be hopeful that whatever age you are, you can opt to enjoy an active sex life, if that suits you, for the rest of your life.

Post-menopausal women are beyond the scope of this discussion on contraception – once you know you are *definitely* unable to get pregnant. This can be hard to establish for certain, though. If a patient wants to stop using contraception, we might look at FSH levels (see Chapters 2 and 3). For example, if you are fifty-one and haven't had a menstrual bleed in over a year and are curious about your contraception status, we might suggest testing the FSH levels to see where you're at. Now, some forms of HRT will artificially reduce your FSH levels and make this method of confirming that you are safe from further pregnancy unreliable, so be forewarned.

If your FSH is elevated, we might repeat the test a few weeks later, just to check it wasn't a fluke or an error – so we can do a blood sample on any given day, and again two to four weeks later. Depending on the level, we might advise that you continue your contraception for another twelve months, just in case. If you don't start getting periods again in that next year, you can stop contraception altogether once the periods are gone and the FSH is persistently elevated. If that's the case, you are now officially 'post-menopausal' and are home free in terms of unexpected pregnancy. It means that your periods are gone and you are probably never going to get pregnant again. If you start getting vaginal bleeding from here on in, you will need to have it thoroughly investigated (as per the previous chapter, it might be related to HRT if you've started on it, or it might be caused by something else).

Aside from tests like FSH, the basic rule of common sense is to use contraception until the age of fifty-five if you are at risk of pregnancy. Typically, pretty much no one gets pregnant without medical assistance after fifty-five years, so it's a reliable cut-off point.

If you are under that age and there is any chance of getting pregnant, you'll want to exercise caution and continue with your chosen contraception method. The ideal contraceptive should be one hundred per cent reliable, convenient, free from side effects, should preserve your future fertility (if applicable), be inexpensive and readily accessible. The famous Professor John Guillebaud, gynaecologist extraordinaire, suggests it should taste like chocolate, too – he gets my vote!

There is no one form of contraception that ticks all these boxes, but many come close. When you seek contraceptive advice, you should be made aware of all the options, the benefits, risks and side effects, and then have an opportunity to make your own informed decision based on your medical needs, restrictions and preferences. *Concordance* is a word used in medical education to describe an approach to health care wherein the patient and the doctor discuss the situation and agree together on a plan. This collaborative approach is key to feeling heard and respected – and you are more likely to be committed to a treatment if you were part of the decision-making process. This is particularly important with contraceptives because their success relies heavily on user compliance. In other words, it can't work if you don't take it or use it.

Your contraception choices

In Europe, we enjoy a fairly comprehensive range of choices (although there are many excellent options that are not yet available in the UK or Ireland). As ever, in terms of HRT, menopause and contraception, the key is finding a combination that suits you. In terms of what you can get your hands on in Ireland and the UK, there are a number of current contraceptive choices. Let's look at each of the options in turn, and then I'll describe them and set out the compatibility of each one with HRT.

Hormonal options

- Combined oestrogen and progestagen products
  - 15 brands of contraceptive pill
  - 1 patch
  - 1 intra-vaginal ring
- Progestagen-only products (POPs)
  - 2 brands of pill
  - 1 intra-muscular injection
  - the single rod or implant known as ImplanonNXT (and as Nexplanon in the UK)
  - 3 intrauterine systems: Mirena, Kyleena and Jaydess
  - 3 types of emergency contraception options, one of which is progestagen hormone-based

Non-hormonal options

- Condoms, male and female
- Diaphragms
- Many and various copper-bearing intrauterine devices or IUDs (copper devices are highly effective emergency contraceptive products, too)
- Sterilization (tubal ligation and vasectomy)
- Natural family planning methods

The pill, patch or ring – how do they work?

Most Europeans who use contraception opt for condoms or the pill. When used correctly and consistently, both of those options provide excellent protection from pregnancy (and, with condoms, sexually transmitted diseases, too). Sadly, though, these options are often used incorrectly or inconsistently, and in such situations the risk of pregnancy is considerably higher. But the pill is reliable if you are reliable in taking it.

Some contraceptive pills contain only progestins (P), some have oestrogen and a progestin (E+P) i.e. the combined oral contraceptive pill (COCP). This combo is also available via a patch or a vaginal ring. There is no oestrogen-only pill because that could cause womb-lining cancer. These products control bleeding more effectively than a progestin-only pill, which is why they are more popular, I think. Unexpected or unusual bleeding is scary to most women and can make some users come off their contraception. There is a risk of blood clots from the oestrogen in the combined pill, so not everyone is allowed to use them. The progestin-only contraceptive pill never causes blood clots.

The combined pill has a strong impact on the hormones in the brain that regulate ovulation. When you take it, it temporarily blocks egg release from the ovaries. It does this through the impact it has on the hypothalamus of your brain. But again, this can only work if you take the pill correctly.

Currently, there are about twenty different brands of combined pill, although some of these are identical preparations made by different companies. In Ireland, there is one combined oestrogen and progestagen hormonal patch, known as Evra. And there is one combined oestrogen vaginal ring, called Nuvaring.

The pill provides contraception and may also give medical benefit for patients with conditions and complaints that are linked to ovulatory dysfunction or menstrual complaints, including dysmenorrhoea (painful periods), menorrhagia (heavy periods), endometriosis (womb-lining tissue in places other than your womb-lining), polycystic ovarian disease (hormone imbalance that can affect ovulation, fertility and more) and premenstrual syndrome.

These powerful artificial hormones have been linked to a variety of serious and some not-so-serious side effects, sadly including venous thromboembolism (blood clots). This means the patient's GP needs to take a careful history and measure her baseline BP and BMI before prescribing the pill. The WHO and the UK's Faculty of Sexual and Reproductive Healthcare (FSRH) have both published guidelines that advise clinicians on the medical eligibility of prospective contraceptive users for all the different types of contraceptive. For example, patients who are living with severe obesity (BMI greater than 39), who are

heavy smokers or who are over fifty years of age are not permitted to
even try the pill (nor, indeed, the patch or vaginal ring) because the
risk of thromboembolism is too high. Basically, to prescribe the pill
for these women would be indefensible.

Minor side effects of the pill, patch and ring are common and include
nausea, headache, sore breasts, mood changes and fluid retention –
very like the typical symptoms of an early pregnancy. These usually
settle on their own if you can bear with them for a month or two, but
a different pill or a completely different contraceptive choice might
eventually be a better option.

The pill, patch or ring – how are they used?

Combined pill users swallow a daily dose of a potent artificial oestrogen (usually ethinyl estradiol) combined with one of a range of
between seven and ten different forms of artificial progestin in varying amounts. The pill hormones cause a temporary anovulation (i.e.
no egg is released, you do not ovulate) in much the same way as pregnancy turns off your ovulations for those nine months. You do not
release eggs when you are pregnant, and you do not release eggs when
you are on the pill. This is a temporary, *healthy* break from monthly
ovulation and does no harm to you or your fertility in the future.

The patch has both oestrogen and progestagen in it, enough to last
seven days. You stick one on your arm or your back, or wherever you
like, and you change it every week for three weeks. Then you take a
break – that is, you do not put a new patch on for a few days. It used
to be recommended that you take a seven-day break, but now we say
only four days. This lets your bleeding kick in and then you start again
on the fifth day with a fresh round of patches.

The ring is a small plastic circle that has three weeks' worth of E+P
inside it. You slide it into your vagina and leave it in there for three
weeks. In that time, you never remove it as there's no need to. It stays
clean and does not interfere with sex or washing. After the three weeks
is up, you take it out and leave it out for four days (again, that used to
be seven) so that your period can kick in. Then on the fifth day you
put in a fresh ring.

The pill *must* be taken every day. But the ring need only be changed once a month and the patch once a week, so either of those might be a better choice for you if you're prone to forgetting to take your pill. The old-style routine of pill taking was to take one every day for three weeks, then come off it for seven days to make a period occur. This is not a natural period. It's just a bleed that happens when contraceptive hormone levels drop, and which doctors call a 'withdrawal bleed'.

We are now being told that this practice is out-dated and may in fact be part of the reason why the pill so often fails. A seven-day break every month might have been advisable fifty years ago, when the pills all had over 100mcg of oestrogen in them, but modern pills are too low dose for that method. People on modern, low-dose pills have been shown to experience ovarian egg activity as early as the fifth day of the seven-day break, which means egg release could start up and pregnancies could occur – especially if you forget to take a pill around the seven-day break. Therefore, doctors are being urged to advise tailored use of the combined pill, patch and ring, recommending their patients skip the seven-day break or take much shorter breaks than recommended on the leaflet that comes in the box. This tailored approach is recommended by the Faculty of Sexual and Reproductive Healthcare (FSRH) – you can ask your doctor or nurse about it.

More and more women are embracing the fact that not having a monthly period while on a contraceptive hormone is healthy and normal and that having a period at all is not necessary. If you do not take these arbitrary breaks off the pill or patch or ring, you won't get that fake period, and that is just fine by most people.

So, what's the twenty-first-century way of taking a combined contraceptive, be it pill, patch or ring? There are three suggested 'tailored use' options.*

- *Option 1: 21/4* – stay on your current brand of pill (or patch or ring), but at the end of every 3 weeks take a 4-day break instead of a 7-day break. This is probably the simplest option. You will still get a light bleed every month, but it will come every 25 days instead of every 28 days. You will be less open to

* These three options are supported by the FSRH, the UK's Royal College of General Practitioners (RCGP) and the World Health Organization (WHO).

an unintended pregnancy, and if you prefer to see a monthly bleed of some kind, well, this will keep it coming. There are apps that help remind you when to stop and restart the pill if you choose the 21/4 option. If you use the patch, wear your 3 patches for the 3 weeks as usual, but stop wearing the patch for 4 days in between each pack instead of 7 days. And for the ring, you wear your ring for 21 days as usual and remove it for 4 days instead of 7 days.

- *Option 2: 63/4* – stay on your current brand but use three packs in a row, i.e. 63 pills/3 rings/9 patches, and then take a 4-day break. You will likely only bleed once every 3 months if you choose this option. This is perfectly healthy, and not only will you be a little more protected against unintended pregnancy, but you will also be spared the pain and hassle of a bleed every month. Again, you will need to track when to take your break and when to restart if you choose this option, or just download one of the free pill-tracking apps.

- *Option 3: 365* – stay on your current pill, patch or ring and use it all the time. This may be the most convenient option for many people as there is no need to set an alarm or keep track of when you need to take a break. If you choose this option, your doctor may suggest that you switch to the lowest-dose version of your pill to reduce the amount of total hormone you are exposed to over time. For example, a patient who uses the 30mg version of a pill and takes it 21 days on/7 days off absorbs more hormone in a year than a patient using the 20mcg version of that same pill but taking it 365 days in a row. The downside to this option is that some users will eventually get some unpredictable vaginal bleeding because the womb-lining has a habit of building up over the months and may need to be allowed to rinse itself out. If you're doing this and you start to bleed for more than 2–3 days in a row, take a break for 4 days, then go right back on the pill where you left off. The upside to this option is better prevention against unintended pregnancy and less pain and hassle from vaginal bleeding. If you use the pill, patch or ring for other reasons, such as PCOS, endometriosis or PMT relief, this may be the best option of all.

Remember: if you have persistent bleeding that does not respond to changing your pill or changing the dose of your pill, you need to contact your doctor as this can also be a sign of infection and other diseases.

What about the pill, patch and ring for women in the menopause?

Okay, after explaining all that, I'm now going to tell you that *you should not be on HRT and the combined pill at the same time*. If you are on HRT and in need of contraception, you could come off the HRT and change to the combined pill/patch/ring, but you cannot use both together. Sometimes, the combined pill is not as good at controlling menopause symptoms, so some people opt to come off it, use a quality HRT and pick another method of contraception.

Sometimes at the clinic we meet POI women who are on the combined pill, say from their GP, and they have read up and know that HRT is, arguably, healthier for POI than the pill because it has better-quality hormones and no associated risk of blood clots with the transdermal oestrogen HRT, but they may need contraception as well. But you *cannot* use the combined pill/patch/ring and HRT – for this contraceptive alone, it is either/or. For all other contraception – mini-pill, injection, bar, condoms, coil, et cetera – you can use them and be on HRT at the same time. But you cannot use the combined contraceptives with HRT.

The mini-pill option

The mini-pill refers to the progestagen-only pill (POP). There is no possibility of life-threatening blood clots with mini-pill use, therefore patients who may have been told not to take the combined pill can usually consider these products. The effectiveness of the mini-pill is approximately the same as the combined pill if used exactly as stated.

In Ireland there are two varieties of progestagen-only contraceptive pills. The modern POPs contain desogestrel and are sold under the names Cerazette and Azalia. We also have an old-fashioned version of the POP which contains norethisterone and is sold as Noriday.

All POPs act by changing the cervical mucus and making it hostile to sperm, but the modern POPs also reliably prevent ovulation. In the UK there is a new POP. This one contains the progestagen drospirenone. It is sold under the name Slinda. It promises to be at least as effective at preventing pregnancies as the desogestrel pills but also to be much better at controlling unexpected bleeding – which is the bugbear of POPs! If it proves to be any good, we'll circle the wagons and see if we can't get Slinda for Irish patients, too.

You may use HRT and the mini-pill at the same time. We cannot assume that the progestagen hormone in your contraception will provide enough hormone to protect the womb-lining from the HRT oestrogen. So, for womb-lining safety, you will need both the progestagen in HRT along with the mini-pill. We regularly recommend those two medications – the mini-pill and HRT – to be used together.

Long-acting reversible contraceptives

The LARC birth control options are very effective and suit many people, especially those who might benefit from a form of contraception that requires less compliance, such as younger people, people who have experienced a failure with the pill in the past, people with disorganized lifestyles, or anyone who craves a simpler life. We can't all be Mary Poppins, so if you're a little less organized than her, you might want to look closely at the LARC options.

These long-acting options are the ones we are encouraged to offer as a first-line option for patients who need high levels of protection but who are not likely to be one hundred per cent accurate with daily pill taking. In terms of presenting an effective contraceptive, it's good to know that pregnancies while using the combined pill are between ten and twenty times more common than failures with a LARC method.

LARC options available in Ireland include:

- Depo-Provera, the only progestagen contraception given by intramuscular injection
- ImplanonNXT, a type of progestagen implant that sits under the skin (some people call it 'the bar')

- Mirena, Kyleena and Jaydess, three progestagen-bearing intrauterine systems
- IUCDs – intrauterine copper devices (popularly known as 'the coil').

Depo-Provera

Depo-Provera is the brand name of one of the most effective forms of contraception, with a failure rate of well under 1 per cent. It contains a synthetic progestagen hormone known as medroxyprogesterone acetate (MPA) that enters the circulation, travels to the brain and causes complete egg release shutdown by blocking the hypothalamus-to-pituitary-to-ovary feedback system. No other form of contraception delivers as much hormone to the blood, which is why it's so reliable. It's pure progestin – no oestrogen in it – and a very potent progestin at that.

Depo-Provera is given as an injection into the arm or bum. It costs approximately €15 privately but is covered by the GMS card. Each injection lasts for more than twelve weeks. (In the UK, however, the licence is fourteen weeks. The discrepancy arises as the company applied for a longer licence in the UK – it's not that something magical happens when you get on the ferry in Holyhead!)

Minor side effects, such as bloating, acne, low mood, irritability and weight gain, can be a problem for some women. Most women notice disruption to their normal monthly bleed, such as extra, unscheduled bleeding (typically in the first three to six months), followed by amenorrhoea, or no periods at all, in the longer term. This amenorrhoea may linger for up to a year or more after the injections are discontinued, so patients planning a baby need to come off it well in advance of trying to get pregnant.

Major side effects are very rare with Depo-Provera. It's a safe option for many who can't use other types of contraception. For example, smokers over the age of thirty-five, overweight people over the age of thirty-five, people suffering from migraine with aura, women who have recently given birth or had a late miscarriage – none of these ladies should be offered any form of combined hormonal contraception (CHC) because the risk of blood clots is so high. However, they can be safely offered Depo-Provera because it does not carry this risk. It can also be used by patients using liver enzyme-inducing medications, without any loss of contraceptive protection.

In fact, Depo-Provera can be used by any patient in almost any situation, although special attention should be paid to people under the age of eighteen and over forty-five. The reason for this is the concern we have about its impact on bone mineral density (BMD). The key hormone in Depo-Provera, MPA, shuts down almost all ovarian activity – and at a brain level, too, not just egg release. When ovarian function is profoundly reduced, less oestrogen is released into the circulation and in some patients this results in a slight drop in BMD. This might not be a problem for everyone, but if you have risk factors for osteoporosis, then maybe Depo-Provera isn't the best option for you, particularly if other options are suitable. You'd need to discuss this clearly with your doctor, check out your osteoporosis risk, and also do a review every two years to check that the Depo-Provera is still suiting you and is still your best option.

You may use HRT and Depo-Provera at the same time – and many women do – but as with the mini-pill we cannot be sure that the progestagen hormone in Depo-Provera will provide enough hormone to protect your womb-lining from the oestrogen in your HRT. You will need both the progestagen in the Depo-Provera for contraception and the progestagen in the HRT for womb-lining safety. This seems a little counter-intuitive to me, as the Depo progestagen is so strong you'd think, how could it *not* protect you from the HRT oestrogen? But at present there are not enough studies to *prove* that it does afford that level of protection. Annoying.

ImplanonNXT (or Nexplanon in the UK) aka 'the bar'

The three-year implant, inserted under the skin of the upper arm, is, statistically speaking, the safest form of contraceptive in the world – even safer than sterilization. Once placed under the skin, the bar allows a 60mcg dose of an artificial progestagen – etonogestrel – to enter the blood circulation every twenty-four hours. The absence of any oestrogen means that people who are prevented from using the combined pill, patch or ring may use the bar safely.

Etonogestrel has a minimal effect on follicle stimulating hormone (FSH) levels and other ovarian function, but still manages to suppress ovulation by means of blocking the luteinizing hormone (LH) surge. While it stops ovulation, this can be reversed within a few days of removing the bar, so return to background fertility is almost immediate.

There are some disadvantages with the bar though. It's tiny and the procedure for inserting it is very easy. But removing it can be tricky, particularly if inserted too deeply into the fascia or muscle. This is why your doctor must be trained in inserting and removing it before performing the procedure. Its removal will cause some scarring.

In terms of the menstrual cycle, the 'low-ish' payload of progestin may result in an erratic and unpredictable bleeding pattern. This is most likely to occur in the first three to six months after insertion and can be controlled, in most cases, with the use of additional hormone. Once the bleeding pattern settles, many people experience no periods at all or just light, acceptable periods. If you continue to bleed erratically, that's a sign to go back to your doctor for some investigations, to find out what's causing the problem, because it might not be the Implanon device.

With the Implanon contraceptive implant or 'bar', about 30 per cent of women do not bleed at all, 30 per cent bleed lightly, and the rest bleed but in an unpredictable way. I think if we could put manners on the bleed patterns, Implanon would win the contraceptive race and the whole world would be getting the bar!

The bar is suitable for use by most people, but the low-dose systemic levels are vulnerable to liver enzyme inducers, so you can't use it with certain anti-epilepsy and tuberculosis drugs, with most HIV retroviral medications, with modafinil ADHD medication (known as Provigil) or with St John's wort, among others.

You may use HRT and the bar at the same time. You will need both the progestagen in the bar for contraception and the progestagen in HRT for womb-lining safety – especially here, as the progestagen in the bar is so gentle that it is unlikely to protect your womb from your HRT oestrogen all on its own.

Intrauterine devices (IUDs)

One of the great things about writing this book is to be able to clear up misinformation – *even among gynaecologists!* This section about hormonal IUDs and HRT is important to me because in my clinic I regularly hear of patients being told the wrong thing, and it drives me nuts. Just the other day, I heard a familiar story: a woman with classic menopause symptoms, who was already well counselled and assessed by her GP, was booked to have a gynaecologist insert a Mirena. The plan was to use the Mirena for the progestagen (and a little contraception) and then start some transdermal oestrogen. The gynaecologist said: *Why would you want to go on HRT if you are still having periods? You are not menopausal yet and, besides, that stuff is dangerous – and it only puts off the inevitable.* I don't know who hurt these doctors, but I do wonder at their amazing ability to talk shite with such authority – please do not comment on topics you know nothing about!

Now for the facts . . .

The basic idea of a hormonal IUD is: instead of delivering contraceptive hormone into the blood circulation, where it travels throughout the system, why not pop it straight into the womb? That is the premise of the three intrauterine systems: Mirena, Kyleena and Jaydess. These hormone-bearing devices are placed at the top of the womb, where they release varying amounts of an artificial progestagen known as levonorgestrel (LNG). They last for six years in the case of Mirena (the licence is seven years in the USA), five years for Kyleena and three years for Jaydess. Although initially expensive for private patients, they will be equivalent to the cost of the pill within twelve to eighteen months. Insertion is usually done while you are awake in the GP surgery or family planning clinic, but they can be inserted under general anaesthetic, if need be.

When it comes to insertion, here is the unvarnished truth: putting them in place might be mildly uncomfortable or wickedly sore. Some people – you carry out the whole procedure and they barely notice the coil going in and are surprised when you tell them you're done. Those are the ones you never hear about! Other people can have terrible experiences. Most women who have had a baby via vaginal delivery can expect a lower degree of cramping/discomfort, but this is by no means a guarantee. Some women who have never had a vaginal delivery, or who had a C-section, might expect to feel a lot of discomfort but then end up getting away with minimal pain – really, it is a roll of the dice. Some may feel faint – indeed, some do actually faint as touching the womb can cause your blood pressure and heart rate to drop. For backup, I suggest that about an hour before the procedure you should take a painkiller of your choice. Personally, I'd opt for ibuprofen, but not everyone can take that.

Whatever way it goes for you, at all times you should be in charge – if you are not happy, tell the doctor, tell them to stop, then you can talk it over and figure it out. And you should check with your doctor beforehand that this stop-and-talk policy *is* their policy – don't allow them to start the process of placing your IUD unless they agree with this approach. Check out the options online before you choose, talk over your choice with your doctor and then, if possible, choose a GP inserter with lots of experience and a smile on their face – or at least a reasonably confident and knowledgeable manner – when they talk to you about the procedure.

In terms of the success and failure rates, it has to be noted that IUDs in general are not as effective as other contraceptive methods at preventing extra-uterine pregnancies. That is to say, they do their best work locally – at the top of the womb, where pregnancies are supposed to stick on and grow. If your pregnancy has decided to stay up in the fallopian tube – known as an ectopic pregnancy – an IUD is less likely to protect you. This is not a common occurrence, but it's necessary to check for an ectopic pregnancy if the IUD doesn't do its job properly. The main cause of a device failing is poor placement technique – another reason to be sure that your doctor has the requisite skill and experience.

Another possible risk of IUDs is that the device could take off on an unplanned journey and perforate the womb muscle. Again, this is rare when it is placed by an experienced inserter, but anyone can be unlucky. These sorts of things are uncommon, but it's as well to know about them, so you have the full picture.

THE MIRENA COIL

You already had me rhapsodizing about the wonders of the Mirena coil in the previous chapter (see pages 158–9). It's an IUD with a 52mg reservoir of the progestin levonorgestrel (LNG). It releases approximately 20mcg of LNG every day over the course of its five-year lifespan (slipping down to 12mcg and 10mcg in the fourth and fifth years, respectively). This alters the cervical mucus, making it spermo-toxic (yep, as it sounds – fatal for the little swimmers), as well as depleting the endometrial lining, which further reduces fertility. Some of the LNG will escape into the blood and in some patients this will result in ovulation ceasing, but this varies from user to user.

As with all such devices, correct placement is essential. You need the insertion to be performed by a doctor who is performing insertions regularly, so they have a high skill level. Removal is usually a much simpler affair and doesn't require formal training. Although there are data to suggest that the contraceptive action of Mirena continues beyond six years, it must be changed after that period if you want to continue to use it as a contraceptive. There is an important exception to this, though: if it was inserted when you were aged over forty-five years, and you've now hit fifty-one with the Mirena still in situ, and you no longer have a natural monthly cycle, you can opt to keep that current device for another five years because your age means a pregnancy is unlikely.

The endometrial depletion that results from local LNG can be so profound that Mirena can also be used to control regular, non-sinister, heavy menstrual bleeding (HMB). If you suffer with HMB and you get relief from those symptoms while wearing a Mirena, and if you are *not relying on it for contraception*, then you could also continue with that current device well past the six-year contraceptive lifespan. But if your menstrual bleeds get heavy again, or if you need contraception as a priority, then you'll need a new device, pronto.

Mirena offers endometrial protection from the effects of HRT oestrogen because the artificial progestin LNG blocks the thickening of the lining layers of the womb that oestrogen can cause. LNG progestin also stabilizes the cells, so they are less likely to undergo changes in their nuclei that can lead to womb-lining cancer.

KYLEENA

A smaller-framed intrauterine system (IUS) was launched in Ireland in 2017. Kyleena has a much thinner frame than its big sister, Mirena, but with a 19.5mg levonorgestrel (LNG) payload coming off it in year one, it gives contraceptive protection for five years. This somewhat lower loading dose is less likely to create full cessation of periods, as Mirena commonly does, and so Kyleena might not be as useful in the treatment of prolonged or heavy menstrual bleeding and has no licence for that as yet. But for younger women, or women who haven't ever given birth, or who have given birth by C-section only, the smaller frame of the Kyleena might fit them better.

You can use HRT and Kyleena at the same time. However, the lower release rate of LNG will not guarantee adequate endometrial protection against HRT oestrogen. This means you'll need progestagen in your HRT as well, to provide adequate protection for your womb-lining.

JAYDESS

Mirena has another littler sister, called Jaydess. It houses only a three-year reservoir of LNG and comes on the same small frame as Kyleena. It is easier and more comfortable to insert, in most cases, than Mirena. Like Kyleena, it allows less LNG to escape from its rate-limiting membrane and so it is licensed for contraception only. It has no application in the treatment of menorrhagia or as endometrial protection in HRT oestrogen users.

The same rules as the previous two IUDs apply if you're on HRT. You can use Jaydess while on HRT, but you'll need progestagen in your HRT to ensure you have adequate protection for your womb-lining.

Intrauterine copper devices (IUCDs), known as 'the coil'

Before explaining the science, I want to share my favourite story about the coil. As many readers will know, artificial forms of contraception are considered sinful by the Catholic Church – we can rely on the rhythm method,* if we choose, but not condoms, diaphragms, coils or hormones. Of course, lots of Catholics wisely ignore the clergy when it comes to their reproductive health, myself included. Now, back in the 1990s when I was working in a family planning clinic, I noticed that every April lady after lady from the travelling community would arrive in to have her copper contraceptive coil removed, only to pop back in at the end of May or early June to have a fresh one inserted. I used to tell them it was a waste of money: *You don't need to do that. Those big copper coils work for 10 years or more!* The penny finally dropped: if they had a child making their First Holy Communion or Confirmation, they did not want to go to Mass and receive Communion with the coils on board. Technically, in that moment, they weren't committing any sin. I love women!

Copper IUDs have been used for generations, with great effect. Copper is both spermo- and ovo-toxic, which means it creates a toxic environment that neither sperm nor eggs want to live in, and it also causes a profound change in the cellular make-up of the endometrium. It doesn't expose the wearer to any form of hormone, but it does give excellent contraception and will last for five, ten or twelve years (or more, depending on the variety). In general, if you have one of the larger coils fitted after the age of forty years, the FSRH suggests it may be left in situ for more than ten years, or until post-menopause is confirmed.

The devices are relatively inexpensive (currently *c.* €25–30 each), making them one of the most cost-effective LARC options. There are hundreds of varieties available worldwide. The FSRH tells us doctors that we should only use devices about which good data exist – which is just common sense. Commonly used copper IUD brands include the CuT380A (the grandmother, the largest of the devices with the greatest amount of data), the TT380 Slimline and Mini TT380 Slimline

---

* The rhythm method is a form of natural family planning. Women must closely track their body temperature and changes in their cervical mucus to work out the best times to have sex, depending on whether they're trying to conceive or avoid conceiving. It's complicated, obviously, and not for everybody and therefore, relative to other forms of contraception, it has a high failure rate.

(don't be fooled, they are both pretty chunky), and the smaller Nova T, which we favour for young people or women who have smaller wombs as they are much kinder to insert.

The coil is efficient and largely reliable once inserted correctly, but one disadvantage is the possible local effect that copper may have on the endometrium, which can cause periods to last slightly longer and become slightly heavier (unlike Mirena, Kyleena or Jaydess). Please note that you always bleed monthly with a coil – if you don't, do a pregnancy test.

We can access a wide variety of IUCDs in Ireland, but these must be sourced by the GP, family planning clinic or a pharmacist, as none of these devices has an Irish distributor at the moment. However, the end of 2022 should see the launch of the version with a specific Irish licence. It will trade under the name Ballerine. The great news is that Ballerine will become the first, and for now only, IUCD covered by the medical card, coming under both the GMS and the Drugs Payment schemes.

Many women opt for HRT alongside their copper coil. As there is no hormone of any kind in the copper coil, you'll need both oestrogen and progestagen in your HRT.

Non-hormonal contraception

If non-hormonal contraception is your preferred option, alongside the copper coil devices there are also various fertility-awareness methods of contraception (for example, the rhythm method) that can be used in conjunction with abstinence or with barrier contraception, i.e. male condom or the female condom, Femidom. There's also a one-size-fits-all silicone diaphragm, known as Caya, which you insert and remove as needed. You can ask your doctor about any of these methods.

In terms of surgical intervention, there's also tubal ligation (under general anaesthetic) for anyone with a uterus – which means getting your tubes tied or clipped.

There are also contraceptives you use after sex that will reduce your risk of conception. There are three different post-coital contraception pills available in Ireland: pills that contain the progestagen hormone levonorgestrel (brand names Norlevo/ Prevenelle) and a pill that contains a progestagen blocker known as ulipristal acetate (brand name ellaOne). These are usually available directly from the pharmacy without a doctor's prescription. Their effectiveness will depend on how likely the episode of sex was to expose you to pregnancy and how soon after the episode of sex you swallow the pill. So, if you think you might need the morning-after pill, get to the pharmacy as quickly as possible.

When any of the copper IUDs are placed after unprotected sex they offer the most effective post-coital contraception of all, but obviously this is lots fussier as you need to find a clinic that offers emergency copper coils (try a family planning clinic) and then pay for the device and the procedure. The upside here is that you may choose to keep the device inside you for the next few years, thereby saving you the hassle of needing emergency contraception again!

KEY TAKEAWAYS

- When comparing contraceptive reliability, the most effective options are either abstinence, sterilization or one of the many LARC options.
- The best form of contraception for YOU is the one that you have chosen and are keen to use.
- HRT is safe to use alongside most forms of contraception – apart from the combined hormonal contraceptive pill, patch or ring. You cannot use HRT and combined contraception products at the same time.
- You must check that your HRT cocktail provides exactly what you need in terms of having enough progestagen to protect your womb-lining from the oestrogen in your HRT.
- Note that by the time this book is published, all of the contraceptives listed here will be free in Ireland for everyone aged seventeen to twenty-five.

PART III

Looking after your heart, breast and bone health during menopause and beyond

17. Your heart and the menopause

Women tend to be extremely aware of the risk of breast cancer and often very concerned about it, but it seems the risk posed by coronary heart disease has slipped under the radar and not really registered for many people. This is unfortunate as heart attack and stroke are among the most common causes of death and illness in older people worldwide. In Ireland, heart disease comes a close second to cancers as a leading cause of death, with approximately 5,000 women dying from cardiovascular disease in 2018 (mainly in the 65+ age group). Thankfully, that number has been coming down for the last five decades as a result of people becoming more health conscious and with the availability of fabulous new treatments for those at risk of heart disease.

The comparison with deaths from breast cancer is striking: 800 Irish women died from breast cancer in 2018. *So, you are nearly seven times more likely to die from heart disease than breast cancer.* You need to let that sink in: talk about a silent killer in our midst – it's like we're all looking in the opposite direction while the Grim Reaper strolls up behind us, whistling. And yet, any doctor or researcher will tell you that fear of breast cancer tops the tables when women are asked about their health concerns and that, when surveyed, most women are far more worried about getting breast cancer than getting heart disease. I wonder why that is? Is it because breast cancer treatments look awful compared to heart disease treatments? Is it because they might take your breast away when you get cancer, but you get to keep your heart? Or is it because it is mostly older women who die from heart disease and part of us thinks, *Oh well, she was a good age*? But then, that is relative – especially as we get older ourselves!

So, let's look squarely at the reality: coronary heart disease is the leading cause of death in women over sixty. Younger women, women with functioning ovaries, are less likely to get heart disease before the menopause compared to men of the same age. However, we know that protection is quickly lost when we go into menopause and our ovaries fail. The cardiac protection that younger women enjoy may have a lot to answer for, as people and health-care professionals seem to think of heart disease – especially cardiovascular diseases like angina and heart attacks – as a 'man's disease'. It isn't.

Heart disease is a woman's disease, particularly as we move into menopause. Therefore, we need to be just as aware of our women's hearts as men should be of their hearts – and so should our doctors. Not only do women lose heart disease protection after the menopause, but our risk of heart attack also catches up with our male counterparts. We might be even more likely than men to die from cardiovascular disease as heart attacks don't always cause the same symptoms in women as in men, and as a result women may not get diagnosed as quickly. Women in the USA, for example, are more likely to die in the first month after a heart attack compared with men, and it's thought this is down to the fact that they receive diagnosis and treatment more slowly than men do. I encountered this very problem recently with a patient at my clinic. She told me how she had presented in A&E with central chest pain that was moving to her left arm and jaw, along with nausea. Her ECG did not display the classic male changes that say 'heart attack'. The staff told her that she was fine and were preparing to send her off home. She was not fine. She ended up going home with two stents inserted. The fact is that heart attacks with normal ECG are more common in women – but still so easily missed.

I have read that in the year after a heart attack, about 25 per cent of men and 38 per cent of women will die from the disease. That's a pretty stark disparity. Part of this disconnect may be because most high-quality studies (randomized control trials) on heart disease have been carried out with male participants only. Women are grossly under-represented in heart disease research (so too are non-Caucasian people), so lots of information we quote about heart disease is based solely on studies involving Caucasian men. Nuff said!

The different kinds of heart and circulation disease

Okay, I know I have to nail down some definitions and explanations here, but I'm not going to lie – it's messy and hard to simplify. But I'll take you through what you really need to know about the diseases themselves, the common acronyms and their definitions, and then we'll look at it through the menopause lens for specific information relating to our mid-life risks.

First off, 'heart disease' is too general a term – it is an umbrella term for diseases of the heart. You can be born with heart disease, you can get it from infections (like Covid-19), you can get it as you age from a combination of genetics and certain unfortunate lifestyle choices – mainly smoking, drinking and being sedentary – and you can get heart disease from parasites. So, lots of ways to get heart disease.

For our purposes, a better term might be cardiovascular disease (CVD), which refers to diseases specific to the blood vessels that supply the heart muscle, and which stem from blockages that prevent or affect the flow of oxygen-rich blood as it moves around the heart muscle. 'Cardiovascular' refers to the blood vessels that supply the muscle of the heart as well as the big momma artery coming out of the heart – the aorta. So, CVD covers lots of common illnesses, like high blood pressure, heart attacks, strokes, angina – that kind of thing. CVD includes:

- *Coronary heart disease (CHD)*: aka coronary artery disease, this is when the main arteries that supply your heart become clogged. They can get partially or completely blocked and can no longer deliver oxygen to specific areas of your heart muscle.
- *Ischemic heart disease (IHD)*: another name for coronary artery disease. It covers the diseases that cause restriction of blood flow within the arteries of the heart, either by blockages or spasm.
- *Heart attack*: crushing or tight chest pain/indigestion/shortness of breath/dizziness caused by extended lack of oxygen to a part of the muscles of the heart. There is irreversible muscle

death in this situation, and if an extensive amount of the heart muscle is affected, it can cause sudden death. The left anterior descending (LAD) artery to the heart supplies a large patch of heart muscle. When it gets fully blocked, as it often does, it's likely the heart will not be able to function efficiently any more. A blockage of the LAD artery is known as 'the widow-maker'. Heart attack is also called a myocardial infarction (MI).

- *Angina* : chest pain/tightness caused by temporary lack of oxygen to a part of the muscles of the heart. The heart muscle is not dead, but oxygen is depleted. This may eventually develop into a heart attack.

- *Cerebro-vascular disease* : a disease of the blood vessels supplying the brain. This is the one we talk about most with regard to HRT as this category of disease can be prevented by early use of HRT.

- *Atherosclerosis* : the process of plaque formation in your artery walls. As we age there is a tendency for the arteries that supply oxygen to the muscles of the heart to get clogged up. *Sclerosis* means when something hardens and *atheroma* is from a Greek word meaning 'gruel' (don't ask me!). Clearly, if the inside of the arteries that bring oxygen-rich blood to your heart get filled with hardened gruel, you are in trouble. The plaques are usually made mainly of certain types of cholesterol.

  This hardening of the arteries is the most common CVD disease and it accumulates slowly over the years. The fatty deposits that build up in the arteries finally lead to a heart attack or stroke. It's not an overnight thing, there will often have been warning signs, there might have been some dodgy lifestyle choices, there may be weight issues and/or obesity, there could well be a family history that links you directly to higher risk. It's a huge problem for women and their doctors, and awareness is key, so that you know what to look for and how to try to prevent it.

- *Transient ischemic attacks (TIAs)* : the supply of oxygen-rich blood to your brain is interrupted temporarily, causing damage to some of the brain cells in that area. Symptoms will vary depending on which part of the brain is affected.

The symptoms of a TIA are just like those of a stroke: facial weakness, changes in your speech, weakness in your limbs, confusion, et cetera, and they require urgent hospital care. You need to be investigated to establish what the cause of your TIA was and be referred for urgent medical intervention. TIAs should *never* be dismissed. Sometimes a blockage is found in one or other of your carotid arteries and can be removed or bypassed to reduce your risk of further TIAs or, worse yet, full stroke.

- *Stroke*: the supply of oxygen-rich blood to your brain is interrupted, causing death of some of the brain cells in that area. Symptoms will vary depending on which part of the brain is affected, but drooping of the face muscles, weakness in the arms, slurred speech and confusion are all common. (You can have bleeding strokes, too. We call them haemorrhagic stroke – like when an aneurysm pops or you fall and injure a brain blood vessel. Haemorrhagic strokes are not associated with the menopause or HRT, as far as we know.)

  Your risk of stroke is lower than your risk of ischemic heart disease, but it's still fairly high – one in five people will experience stroke in their lifetime. The key indicator for stroke is high blood pressure (BP), so again you're back to healthy lifestyle choices and monitoring in order to maintain healthy blood pressure. I mean, that's the good news here – there's lots you can do yourself to protect your heart, brain and the rest of your body. I hope that everyone knows they need to get their BP checked from time to time after they hit the age range of forty-five to fifty as it can be well elevated *with no symptoms*.

- *Deep vein thrombosis and pulmonary embolism*: blood clots in the leg veins, which can dislodge and move to the brain, heart and lungs.

- *Peripheral arterial disease*: the supply of oxygen-rich blood to your legs is blocked. This can cause cramping leg pain on exercise, which is usually relieved by rest, but it can progress to severe blockage, with gangrene and amputation in some cases.

- *Rheumatic heart disease*: damage caused to the heart muscle and heart valves by rheumatic fever.

- *Congenital heart disease*: birth defects that affect the normal development and functioning of the heart.
- *Atypical types of heart-related diseases*: in addition, women are more likely to get other unusual types of heart-related diseases, such as:
  - a coronary spasm – this is when one of the blood vessels that supplies oxygen to your heart muscle clamps down and mimics a heart attack
  - a coronary dissection or spontaneous coronary artery dissection (SCAD) – this is when the wall of one of the blood vessels supplying oxygen to your heart tears
  - takotsubo cardiomyopathy – this is an inflammatory reaction where the heart muscle enlarges, and it often happens after being subjected to emotional stress. This is why they sometimes call it Broken Heart Syndrome!

Women's experience of angina and heart attacks

A heart attack may not feel the same for a woman as it does for a man. Men typically present to the surgery or hospital with chest pressure – 'I feel like an elephant is sitting on my chest,' they may say. The chest pain/pressure classically radiates or moves down the left arm or into the left jaw, according to my old textbooks. Women can also experience chest pressure, and it is the most common symptom, but they are more likely to say they are also experiencing nausea and/or vomiting, shortness of breath, fatigue, sweating, feeling light-headed or dizzy – and, of course, we may feel pain in the neck, jaw, throat, abdomen or back.

As I mentioned already, a big problem for women is the response we receive when we complain of what might be CVD. If a man is being investigated for a suspected heart attack, one of the blood tests carried out is for the presence of cardiac troponins, which are proteins that are released from damaged heart muscle. The levels of these proteins that are used to rule out heart attack are based on studies in men – which means mild elevations of cardiac troponins in women having heart attacks could be missed. There should be adjustments made to those results when treating women.

Also, the gold standard screening test for atherosclerosis is cardiac catheterization and dye. This is where they take X-ray videos of the blood swooshing around your heart blood vessels through use of a dye injected into your wrist. However, this test looks for blockages in large arteries, yet we know women are more likely to get atheroma in the smallest arteries of the heart, which again means a diagnosis could be missed.

Heart tests that might be more appropriate for women include a cardiac MRI, which can identify inflammation of the heart, and an electrocardiograph (ECG). You will know the ECG monitor well from every medical drama you have ever watched on TV. That will be the screen showing lines jumping up and down, making a regular or irregular beeping noise as the heart beats. And then goes *booooooooooooooooooooooo* and the lines stop moving when the medics turn off life support – the origin of the term 'flatlined', meaning that some-one has died. The ECG is an essential tool in diagnosing heart disease events like heart attacks. The lines on the screen trace the electrical signals moving through your heart muscles. There are a few changes to the waves on an ECG reading that might alert us to a heart attack. For instance, some of the waves usually become elevated when heart muscle has died as a result of a heart attack and the electrical pathways through heart muscle have to be 'rerouted'.

Some people get what are called non-STEMI heart attacks. ST is the segment of the ECG reading related to heart attacks, so a non-STEMI heart attack means there's no alarming elevation in the ST segment in this MI. This is what happened to my lady in the story above – when she went to A&E but they couldn't detect her heart attack. Women may be more likely to have a non-STEMI than men, and even though we might have heart disease risks, women with non-STEMI are sometimes treated less aggressively than men – we pull out all the stops if a man has chest pain, while sometimes telling a lady to see her GP about anxiety medication!

Why do women get more heart disease after menopause?

Women are less likely to have heart disease before the menopause than men of the same age, but that protection is lost when our ovaries slow down. Like so many diseases that seem to get up a head of steam once we lose our main ovary hormone, estradiol, our heart disease risk climbs quickly after the ovaries start to fail. This is borne out by the fact that CVD is less common in younger women than in older women, and research suggests that this is to do with the many cardio-vascular benefits given to us by oestrogen.

It has been suggested that menopausal women who get severe or persistent hot flushes may be at higher risk of heart disease. Women reporting more frequent or more severe hot flushes seem more likely to have more plaque and increased carotid intima-media thickness (CIMT). What does that mouthful mean? Well, the arteries from your heart leading up to your brain are called the carotids. They are subject to clogging, too, and we can measure the development of carotid plaque formation via ultrasound scans. Higher levels of carotid thickness are a predictor of *silent atherosclerosis*, which could impact you later. Measuring CIMT is easily done and not invasive, as opposed to, say, an angiogram (the dye into the heart), where rare but life-threatening complications could occur. That said, such complications are rare and the angiogram is the gold standard test, so if you need it, go get an angiogram.

So, if you have a family history of heart disease, if you have been a smoker, or sedentary, or have bad lipids, or blood pressure, or all of the above, you need to make some time to get a check-up and ask your GP specifically about heart health investigations.

HRT and heart disease – the good and not-so-good news

I'll cut to the chase here: HRT can be protective, but once you have heart disease, it's not a treatment. Some research has suggested that HRT use seems to reduce the risk of heart disease and can protect women against it developing. This depends on several factors. And here we need to make a very important distinction: all HRT is not the same and all oestrogens are not the same.

Most of the research (and there is actually not much) done in the last forty years looking at HRT use and what effect it might have on heart disease in women was carried out on women who were using equine oestrogens and the relatively strong progestagen MPA. The studies looked at women who were much, much older than the age at which women typically start using HRT today, which meant that for many of the women involved, heart disease would have already taken hold. (Remember that the Women's Health Initiative (WHI) accepted women as old as seventy-nine into its study.) While MPA is a good progestagen for preventing pregnancy, and really useful in stopping unexpected bleeding on HRT, it is possible that even greater heart protection and benefits could be gained from using HRT that offers bio-identical human oestrogen (no horse's wee, thank you) and gentler bio-identical progestagens, such as P4. However, the studies on those products and their impact on women as we age are only being done now, so the jury is still out.

As mentioned above, there is a tendency for the arteries that supply oxygen to the muscles of the heart to get clogged up as we age (atherosclerosis). The blockages that accumulate in our heart arteries are made up of fat, cholesterol, calcium, waste products from dead cells, and a clotting agent called fibrin. The plaques start to slowly build up from the time we are kids and, depending on our genes, lifestyle habits, other diseases we might have, and sometimes just bad luck, they can get so large that they start to block blood flow to the muscles of the heart, causing angina or a full-blown heart attack.

Sometimes, tiny pieces of these plaques can crack off (embolize) and travel to either another part of the heart or to our brain blood vessels, causing a stroke. The science of why these plaques develop, and how we can slow them down, is complex, but one thing we all agree on is that most oestrogen – especially bio-identical oestrogen – helps delay plaque formation. The oestrogen won't fix the plaques once they are already in there, however, so it is not a treatment for atherosclerosis – it is a prevention. So, early intervention to maintain oestrogen levels and prevent plaques building up is key – especially in women who go through premature ovary hormone loss, because they have a higher risk of developing oestrogen deficiency diseases, like heart disease.

Only two large-scale studies are available to tell us about women's heart disease and HRT: the less than helpful WHI study (first results published in 2002; see Chapter 9) and the Nurses' Health Study (first results published in 1998). Both showed that women were given some protection by HRT if they started it close to the age of their last menstrual period. These studies also warned us to be careful with the dose of oestrogen – bigger doses may destabilize coronary plaques. The women in the WHI study were using oral equine oestrogen HRT, which we know increases thrombosis risk and may precipitate a stroke or heart attack if given to women who already have hardening of the arteries. So that doesn't reflect modern HRT usage. The WHI participants were also on the potent artificial progestagen MPA (aka Provera), which is used widely in contraception, period control and many forms of HRT. It is possible that some of the unhelpful impact of HRT on vessel disease had as much to do with the progestagen used in those older studies as with the oestrogen used, and also the age at which the patient started her HRT. Certain progestagens do appear to work against the benefits of the HRT oestrogen, particularly MPA, so we need to be cautious with progestagen choices.

A French study from about ten years ago linked having higher blood levels of oestrogen to a greater risk of heart disease. Uh oh, did we have it wrong? we asked ourselves. Does keeping our oestrogen levels higher with HRT actually increase our risk of heart disease?

The answer is no.

Most of the French women in that study were not on HRT. The ladies who were found to have the higher oestrogen levels in their blood probably had elevated amounts of E1 (estrone) as that is the main oestrogen left over after your ovaries stop making E2 (estradiol). We know women living with overweight and obesity have more estrone in their body because it is made in fat cells . . . you can see where this is going!

At present there are no large trials or prospective studies looking at the different effects on heart disease we might see when using modern, low-dose, bio-identical, transdermal oestrogen versus oral estradiol versus oral equine oestrogen versus nothing. We only have small 'look back' studies, known as observational studies. We really need those large prospective studies to be carried out.

In the meantime, when our patients on HRT start moving into their sixties and beyond, we usually suggest they alter their HRT products to keep away from oral oestrogen of any kind (to avoid increased risk of clots) and switch from stronger progestagens to something gentler, like P4 (micronized progesterone). This will depend to some degree on your own preferences, but why not opt for the products that are thought to be best for your heart as you age? When I talk about the HRT benefits to the heart in this book, and when I prescribe HRT with a view to a healthy heart, I am talking only about bio-identical HRT – the good stuff. I'm talking about the 17-beta estradiol that you take in through the skin and the micronized progesterone (Utrogestan) that you can swallow or insert vaginally.

The benefit of HRT for heart health all depends on timing

In 2019 the British Menopause Society (BMS) released a Consensus Statement on the role of HRT in the prevention of heart disease in younger menopausal women. This quotes a 2012 Danish study, reported in the *British Medical Journal*, which involved about two thousand Danish women, with an average age of fifty, who were given either a placebo (about a thousand of the participants), 2mg of oral estradiol on its own if they'd had a hysterectomy (very few ladies were in this group), or 2mg/1mg of oral estradiol with 1mg of NET progestagen if they had a womb (about a hundred participants). They concluded that after ten years of treatment, women receiving the oral HRT soon after their last period had a significantly reduced risk of mortality, heart failure or heart attack.

Interestingly, they did not notice any apparent increase in risk of cancer, blood clots or stroke. The study authors compared this information to the less favourable heart outcomes of the WHI study, in which the average age of those women was sixty-four years and the HRT used was oral equine oestrogen – in a pretty high dose for an older woman – along with a high dose of the artificial progestagen MPA.

Based on all of this information, researchers have come up with the Timing Hypothesis of HRT. That is, that early use of certain types of HRT is heart healthy, while delayed or later use of HRT probably won't protect your heart at all. If you keep the doses low and use transdermal oestrogen and bio-identical progesterone, it probably won't do any harm, *but* you need to get your cardiovascular system as healthy as you can at the same time.

The BMS says: 'No reductions, but also no increases, were shown in women starting HRT after 60 years or beyond 10 years post-menopausal.' This is a really important point as it means you can try HRT for symptom relief if you are over sixty, but the potential for that HRT to protect you from heart disease is probably gone.

And what about when you come off HRT? After the WHI study was prematurely discontinued, there seemed to be an uptick in heart disease and stroke in the group of women using the real HRT (as opposed to the placebo), which gave us all a bit of a fright and suggested women ought to be very gradual about stopping their hormones if they had a choice. A more recent Finnish study tells us that this phenomenon is unlikely if HRT is discontinued after the age of sixty.

What effect does HRT have on the heart?

We're going back to atherosclerosis here, to look at what HRT oestrogen might be able to do about it.

As we already said, atherosclerosis is the term used to describe the complex lumps of material that start to clog up our arteries as we age. Pieces can travel off and block a smaller artery, and maybe cause a heart attack or a stroke. Autopsies have revealed plaques in the arteries of people as young as fifteen years of age in the USA. It probably happens here in Ireland, too. It is more common to start to develop these lesions young if you smoke, have high blood pressure and/or are overweight or are genetically predisposed to it. So, heart disease starts early, but you can always do something to slow it down and even reverse it.

Estradiol protects younger women from the development of atheroma plaques by lowering the amount of lipid deposits in the blood vessel wall. But atheroma plaques become more common in the arteries

of our hearts as we hit the perimenopause, between the ages of forty
and fifty, and then we see a big increase in atheroma after fifty years
of age for women who are not on HRT. We all have them, but most
are pretty small and don't cause us trouble. But we are likely to get
symptoms from the vessel disease by the time we are sixty-five.

Unfortunately, if an atheroma is *already* in the blood vessel, giving
estradiol via HRT – especially a high dose oral HRT – may cause
a plaque to break up and travel. It's a case of estradiol being good in
healthy blood vessels, to keep them healthy, but posing a risk to existing atheroma plaques in the blood vessels, particularly at high doses.

So, you can see it's all about timing. This underlies the thinking that
early introduction of estradiol via HRT can prevent vessel disease in
women with generally healthy vessels but, sadly, could precipitate a
heart attack or a stroke in a patient who already has significantly dis-
eased vessels.

Now you're probably wondering: so how can I check my level of
atheroma in order to inform my decision whether to take HRT or
not? We assume that healthy women who are low risk, have no symptoms and are under fifty-five to sixty years of age are unlikely to have
critical narrowing. Anyone else we can refer for thorough testing.

Ovarian oestrogen can also improve the functions of the inner walls
of the blood vessels that supply blood to the heart. The inner layers of
those blood vessels – the endothelial layers – get stiff and less supple
with prolonged oestrogen loss. Even when you give them the oestrogen back, if it has been too long the blood vessels will not only derive
no benefit from that oestrogen, but it could cause a clot or narrowing of the vessel.

Ovarian oestrogen also affects smooth muscle, which is the type of
muscle found in the walls of our blood vessels. Oestrogen seems to
stop those muscles from constricting, thereby keeping the blood flow
to the heart as free-flowing as it can be. And maintaining oestrogen
levels in the blood also seems to slow down or prevent thickening of
the carotid arteries between your heart and your brain, another cause
of heart disease after menopause.

As for progestagen, the key thing to note is that just as with oestrogen not all progestagens are the same. Some progestagens, especially
natural ovarian progestagen – which is available in HRT as micronized

progesterone (P4) – have been shown to prevent atheroma plaque formation, just as oestrogen does. Micronized progesterone decreases bad cholesterol (LDL) and increases good cholesterol (HDL).

What you can do for your heart

The World Health Organization (WHO) tells us that 80 per cent of heart disease can be prevented by diet and lifestyle changes. Welcome to your Modifiable Risk Factors!

Blood pressure (BP)

This tends to climb after menopause, with about one-third to half of all women having high BP or raised normal BP after their final period. Incidentally, high BP after menopause is more common in women who had BP problems when pregnant. Hypertension is a silent problem at first, and you may go years with high blood pressure without realizing it. The most recent recommendations for assessing BP – which your GP will likely follow – is to ask you to buy a home BP monitor and do a series of home readings at different times throughout the day, note them down, and bring that information to your GP.

If you are diagnosed with high BP, get on treatment. You may need to work this out over months with your GP because not everyone is suited to the same BP therapies, but keep at it and don't stop the tablets just because 'I feel fine'. Famous last words!

High blood pressure is one of the most correctable risk factors for heart attacks and strokes. Transdermal oestrogen tends to lower the systolic blood pressure (the top number), but some types of oral oestrogen (especially equine oestrogen) can increase it. So, get your BP checked and corrected, if need be. You can safely use transdermal oestrogen and BP medicine together.

Smoking

I know smokers hate to hear it, but **don't smoke**. You are six times more likely to have a heart attack if you smoke more than twenty cigarettes a day. One year after stopping, that risk is halved, and it continues to drop with time. Don't start smoking if you haven't already. If you're a smoker, cut down. If you find it hard to cut down, get some nicotine replacement help because it significantly improves your chances of staying off cigarettes. See the HSE's website www.quit.ie for help.

Diabetes

Women with diabetes appear to have a higher risk of cardiovascular disease than men with diabetes, according to the BMS. Using HRT, particularly transdermal oestrogen and non-androgenic progestagen, may decrease the risk of type 2 diabetes and improve insulin metabolism.

Overweight/obesity

Obesity, in particular central or abdominal obesity, which is when your waist measures more than 88cm, is linked to increased risk of cardiovascular disease. Your risk is much higher as a woman if you also have any one of these: high triglycerides, low HDLs, high BP, diabetes or pre-diabetes. Ask your GP for help as we are now learning to consider overweight and obesity as a chronic health disease instead of a sign of your bad eating choices. Help is out there.

Abnormal lipids

Too much bad cholesterol or too little good cholesterol can start to become a problem after menopause. I already discussed cholesterol in Chapter 8. Cholesterol is an essential molecule that is found in every cell in the body. We use it to make hormones like oestrogen, progesterone and vitamin D. We also use it to make bile acids in the liver, which will absorb fats during digestion. So, we need some cholesterol, but not too much. We certainly don't need too much of the less helpful types of cholesterol. Why? Because the bad cholesterol can find its way into your arteries and will speed up atheroma development, which is, of course, the main cause of heart attacks, strokes and other vessel disease. High levels of bad cholesterol – LDLs (low density lipoproteins) – and of TGL (triglycerides) have been linked to a greater risk of heart disease. High density lipoproteins (HDLs) are heart healthy and can help balance out abnormally high LDLs or TGLs. Oral oestrogen reduces LDLs and increases HDLs, but they also increase TGLs. Androgenic progestagens (LNG and NET) can reduce HDLs, so talking to your doctor about the choice of progestagen in your HRT – like micronized progesterone (P4) – would be wise if you suffer with abnormal lipids.

Alcohol

Epidemiological studies show that low alcohol consumption has a beneficial effect on cardiovascular disease. But heavy drinking, and especially episodic binging, can have the opposite effect and should be avoided.

Being active

The WHO recommends 150 minutes of moderate activity a week, to reduce the risk of heart disease, obesity and diabetes. Using HRT may aid restful sleep and help to ease joint aches and pain, which might in turn encourage exercise.

KEY TAKEAWAYS

- ☒ Heart disease is just as likely to affect women as men after we enter the menopause.
- ☒ Our genes play a big role in our individual risk, but many other 'modifiable' factors play an important role, and you can do something about those.
- ☒ Be aware of your own risk – maybe try the QRISK®3 calculator: https://qrisk.org/three/.
  Try not to smoke, aim to drink less, be active, eat smart, and get your blood pressure and cholesterol checked regularly.

18. Breast cancer and the menopause

After skin cancer, breast cancer is the second most common cancer in women in Ireland. The likelihood of being diagnosed with breast cancer increases as we age, and 1 in 9 females will be diagnosed with breast cancer in our lifetimes, with most of the diagnoses made in people who are over fifty and post-menopause.

When looking at the risk of breast cancer, we need to consider age. Young people are less likely to be diagnosed with breast cancer, but when it happens, it can be devastating. The risk of being diagnosed with breast cancer tends to go up with age so that by the time you are ninety years old, you have about a 1 in 10 chance of having a breast cancer – although you may never be diagnosed at that age because doctors tend to stop doing mammograms and examining the breasts for women over seventy.

The USA's National Institute of Health publication tells us that the risk of being diagnosed with breast cancer by age is as follows.

- Age 30: 0.49 per cent (or 1 in 204)
- Age 40: 1.55 per cent (or 1 in 65)
- Age 50: 2.40 per cent (or 1 in 42)
- Age 60: 3.54 per cent (or 1 in 28)
- Age 70: 4.09 per cent (or 1 in 24) – this decrease is related to low detection rates rather than a drop in rate of risk

The other thing to be aware of is that when we say 'cancer', this covers a spectrum of disease, some highly survivable, others not so much, sadly. The term 'breast cancer' is really just a blanket term as there are lots of different types of breast cancer – which is the case with all cancers these days. Breast cancers can be aggressive in their growth and the way they spread, or they can be slower in their growth and therefore slower to spread. Some breast cancers can be strongly influenced by hormones, while others might have no hormone receptors on them at all.

Breast cancer has always been thought to be linked to ovarian hormones – particularly oestrogen and progestagen – but exactly what that relationship is and how hormones might affect breast cancer development is quite complicated and not yet fully understood. Over the years, research has suggested that higher hormone levels would likely increase your risk of breast cancer as most breast cancers do have hormone receptors on them. This makes sense – but to what degree? How much of an influence does, say, the use of HRT have on your personal risk of being diagnosed with breast cancer?

Well, no one knew for sure, so in the mid-1990s the now infamous US study on older women and HRT and breast cancer (called the Women's Health Initiative (WHI) – see Chapter 9) started to enrol women into its trial, and in 2002 its first results were published. The WHI study showed that for *most* women between the ages of fifty and sixty (which is the age group where most HRT users reside), the average risk of breast cancer detection (in the USA) was 23 out of 1,000 women. They also found some other factors that seemed to affect the chances of being diagnosed with breast cancer. One of those factors was using HRT.

The WHI found that for the women who were *not* using HRT at all (in the study they gave some women a dummy pill), their risk of breast cancer diagnosis remained the same as the average, i.e. 23 in 1,000.

For those women using the typical oestrogen + progestagen HRT combo (although in this case, they only used horse urine oestrogens and a high-dose artificial progestagen), the risk of being diagnosed with breast cancer increased – not straight away, but after about four years – to 27 in 1,000. That is an important piece of information to take note of and requires further exploration.

The study showed some other interesting trends:

- The women who had their wombs removed were put on plain horse urine oestrogen and their risk of being diagnosed with breast cancer decreased to 19 in 1,000. That was odd!
- The risk of being diagnosed with breast cancer among women who drank more than 2 units of alcohol a day was also higher,

up to 28 in 1,000 – this was higher than the risk seen for the women on the standard HRT combo.

- The risk of being diagnosed with breast cancer among the women who were overweight (BMI above 30, see Chapter 22) was the highest of all, at 47 in 1,000. That's a bit disturbing for overweight people like myself!
- On the positive side, women who exercised more than 2.5 hours a week were far less likely to be diagnosed with breast cancer, at 19 in 1,000.

The WHI study was very valuable in some ways but limited in many others, not least by the fact that only a small number of the women who participated were in the fifty to sixty age bracket. The majority were sixty-three or older, which isn't at all representative of women taking HRT today. But it is instructive nonetheless to see those breast cancer risk factors with regard to alcohol, BMI and exercise. That's important information for any woman because we can do something about those particular risk factors.

A survivable cancer

These days, breast cancer is considered a very survivable cancer, and more and more women will be living with a breast cancer diagnosis than ever before. Every year, around 3,351 Irish women are diagnosed with breast cancer and about 700 women will die from it, but when caught early, breast cancer has a high five-year survival rate (85 per cent). Despite the positive news on survival rates, for many of us breast cancer remains the most frightening cancer to imagine being diagnosed with.

The other thing to say about the 'survival' rates is that there is an argument about the meaning of the statistics. Some experts maintain that as we are diagnosing breast cancers very early, mainly via screening mammography, we may, in fact, be *over-diagnosing* breast cancer. Now, you would naturally think that the earlier you diagnose a cancer, the better, and because it's small it can be treated, or even cured, more readily. Unfortunately, in some situations early screening will identify abnormalities in breast cells that might never have gone on to become cancerous, or very low risk cancers that would never have developed or would have simply disappeared. But once that person is diagnosed with breast cancer and receives treatment, she is now a 'breast cancer survivor' and she must deal with all that implies. Some experts would argue that the over-diagnosis of breast cancer via screening mammography is not actually saving lives per se, but only creating stress for many women and putting them through sometimes unnecessary treatment. I am not an expert on this particular issue. I would take every and all breast cancer therapies offered to me if I were diagnosed as I would be scared to death to do otherwise. But more work needs to be done for women, their vulnerable breasts, and cancer diagnosis and treatment.

That's an argument that will likely rage for some time, but for our purposes it is a fact that breast cancer poses a significant threat to the health and well-being of Irish people not only in the treatment of the disease itself but also in how we manage those people when they enter the perimenopause/menopause. Your breast cancer treatment might tip you into early menopause, for example, and that has to be planned and managed. Even if that doesn't occur, you might be on medication for five to ten years in the aftermath of diagnosis and that will affect your choices in terms of menopause treatment. This is why I'm devoting a separate chapter to breast cancer, because it affects so many of us and in so many ways.

Nonetheless, it must be acknowledged right up front that this is a controversial area, and probably the most difficult chapter to write. I won't be able to provide easy answers, I'm afraid. All I'm aiming to do is to give you the current information from reputable medical sources so that you will be more empowered to make decisions when it comes to your menopausal symptoms, the options you have in managing them and the implications, if any, with regard to your breast cancer risk.

Breast cancer – a term for many different cancers

Breast cancer is an umbrella term for the many different types of malignant cells that can be diagnosed in the breasts of a patient, male or female. There are three main parts to your breasts: the lobules, the ducts and the connective tissue. The lobules produce the milk. The ducts carry the milk to the nipples. The connective tissue (fat cells and fibrous tissue) hold it all together. Breast cancers may arise in any of these areas, although they usually arise in the lobules or the ducts.

The most common form of breast cancer diagnosis is *ductal carcinoma*. These are cancers that start in the milk-producing ducts and they can either stay local, which is known as *ductal carcinoma in situ (DCIS)*, or they can spread to (invade) other tissues, which is known as *invasive* or *infiltrating ductal carcinoma (IDC)*.

IDC can sometimes be found in other parts of the body as the cells can travel through the lymph system or through the bloodstream.

DCIS is a common breast disease diagnosis that is more a pre-cancer than an actual cancer. It might go on to become invasive breast cancer, it might not. In DCIS, the cancer cells are limited to the lining of the ducts only. A biopsy of DCIS may reveal it to be of low, intermediate or high grade. This finding helps predict the likelihood of those cells going on to invade other tissues.

Invasive lobular breast cancer (ILC) is a breast cancer that starts in the milk-producing glands, the lobules. Those cells can spread into the surrounding tissue and sometimes into other parts of the body through the lymph system or through the bloodstream. Alternatively, they can stay put in the lobules of the breast, which is referred to as *lobular carcinoma in situ (LCIS)*. LCIS is not actually a cancer and is usually managed by regular breast exams and mammograms. It is, however, a risk factor for developing invasive breast cancer so treatment may be offered, which will usually be via anti-oestrogen hormonal therapies.

ILCs are more likely to have oestrogen and progestagen receptors (see below) on them than IDCs. They are more likely to be found in older people when compared with IDCs, and are often bigger in size and more likely to have spread outside the breast by the time they are diagnosed. Why this is, we don't know for sure. Maybe they grow more slowly than IDCs? Maybe they are harder to detect on mammogram?

There are also other, less common types of breast cancer that can be diagnosed, including medullary, mucinous, tubular, metaplastic, papillary and inflammatory breast cancer, as well as a condition known as Paget's disease of the nipple. I haven't got the education or the confidence to cover these in detail here.

How different types of breast cancer are classified

In addition to there being different cell types of breast cancer, there are other important distinctions within a breast cancer type, including:

- what *receptors* the cancer cells have on them – meaning its sensitivity to hormones
- what *stage* the cancer is at – this refers to its spread
- what *grade* of cancer you have – this refers to its potential to grow.

Receptors

After a mammogram, you might be told that you need to have a biopsy. This entails taking a piece of tissue and testing it to confirm the presence of cancer cells, where the cancer came from (ducts or lobes) and to discover the hormone status of the tumour: that is, whether the cells have specific receptor sites in them that will be affected by hormones. This means that the cancer cells have a sensitivity to hormones, and that sensitivity can make them receive the hormone into the cell and grow. The main subtypes are:

- oestrogen receptor: + or − (i.e. positive or negative)
- progestagen receptor: + or −
- HER2 receptor: + or −

A *hormone receptor positive breast cancer* can be ER+, PR+ or both ER+ and PR+. The presence of oestrogen and/or progestagen in the body can promote the growth of ER+/PR+ cancer cells. Most breast cancers (about two out of three) will be either ER or PR positive. Less often, breast cancers will be ER and PR negative or hormone receptor negative.

It is standard procedure to offer patients with ER+ or PR+ breast cancer a medical treatment that will either block the ER/PR receptors in your body or reduce the amount of oestrogen or progestagen in your bloodstream. For reasons that will be obvious to you now, these treatments can cause or exacerbate menopausal symptoms.

HER2 is an acronym for Human Epidermal growth factor Receptor 2. It is a protein that can be present on the surface of breast cancer cells. The HER 2 protein can promote the growth of the cancer cells. Only about 15 to 20 per cent of people with breast cancer are HER 2+. Specific drugs are used to treat HER 2+ breast cancer, but those medicines do not usually affect menopause symptoms in themselves.

Triple negative breast cancer is when doctors find neither ER, PR nor HER 2+ receptors in your tumour. This is more common in younger women, with an incidence of about 15 to 20 per cent of people with breast cancer, and is sometimes linked to cancer gene mutations, like BRCA (see pages 218–22).

Staging

Assessing the stage your cancer is at depends on the size of a tumour and whether it has spread or not. The most popular classification method used in Ireland and the UK is the number staging system. The number staging system for breast cancer gives a number value from 1 to 4, depending on where your cancer has been detected.

- *Stage 1A* = the tumour is less than 2cm and no cancer was found in the armpit lymph nodes.
- *Stage 1B* = the tumour is not found in the breast tissue or is < 2cm and micro metastases were found in armpit lymph nodes.
- *Stage 2A* = the tumour is between 2cm and 5cm and has not spread to the armpit lymph nodes OR the tumour was not detected in the breast but was found in 1 to 3 nearby armpit lymph nodes.

- *Stage 2B* = the tumour is between 2cm and 5cm and it has spread to 1 to 3 armpit lymph nodes OR the tumour is > 5cm but has not spread to the armpit lymph nodes.
- *Stage 3* = the tumour is 'locally advanced', that is, it has spread to nearby tissues like the skin of your chest, the armpit lymph nodes and sometimes to nearby other local lymph nodes.
- *Stage 3A* = the tumour is not found in the breast or is < 5 cm but has spread to 4 to 9 armpit lymph nodes OR the tumour is > 5cm and was found in < 3 armpit lymph nodes.
- *Stage 3B* = the tumour has spread to nearby tissues, like the skin of the breast, chest wall and muscle. It may be found in armpit lymph nodes but < 9 of them.
- *Stage 3C* = the tumour has spread to > 10 armpit lymph nodes OR the tumour has spread to nodes under your chest or your neck as well as to > 4 of your armpit lymph nodes.
- *Stage 4* = the tumour has travelled beyond the breast and surrounding tissue to distant areas, usually the bones, liver, lungs.

THE SIGNIFICANCE OF THE LYMPH NODES

The lymph system is like a security system for the body. Lymph is a watery fluid made up of some of the liquid part of what constitutes blood. There are lymph vessels, nodes and glands all over the body and they are designed to do lots of jobs, including keeping the liquid-to-cell ratio of the blood balanced (homeostasis) and protecting us from disease or infection via the action of lymphocytes (white blood cells that are the frontline soldiers in our immune system). The lymphocytes attack germs and try to filter out viruses and bacteria that could threaten the body.

The lymph nodes and lymph travel in parallel to blood circulation. By infiltrating the bloodstream or the lymph system, cancer cells can spread beyond the area where they originated and go to distant parts of the body.

Grading

Establishing the grade of a breast cancer relates to its growth potential. The oncology team looks at the cells under a microscope and compares the speed of growth of the cancer cells to normal cells.

- *Grade 1* = cancer cells appear similar to normal breast cells, also known as 'well differentiated', and they usually grow slowly. They are less likely to spread. Grade 1 is also called *low grade cancer.*
- *Grade 2* = cancer cells appear more abnormal than other breast cells and will grow slightly faster than Grade 1 cells. Grade 2 is also called *moderate* or *intermediate grade cancer.*
- *Grade 3* = cancer cells look much more abnormal than healthy breast cells, often referred to as 'poorly differentiated', and they will grow much more quickly than Grade 1 or 2 cells. Grade 3 is also called *high grade cancer.*

The benefits of screening for breast cancer

When cancer is first diagnosed, often after you or your doctor find a lump, it is usually larger and can be at a more advanced stage because small cancers are hard to feel, especially if your breast connective tissue is dense.

When cancers are detected at a routine mammogram they are usually smaller and at an earlier stage. As I mentioned earlier, this can mean that very low risk cancers are detected that would possibly have gone away all by themselves, without diagnosis or treatment. Over-diagnosis is a problem for health scientists in all areas of health care and is also an issue for breast cancer doctors and their patients.

An additional problem with the current forms of breast cancer screening is *false positives*. Just as a mammogram X-ray can miss a breast cancer (because no screening test is one hundred per cent guaranteed), it can also detect something in a breast that starts a whole chain-reaction of further investigations, procedures, and the anxiety associated with all that, only to discover there was nothing wrong with you in the first place. Therefore, breast screening should not be recommended indiscriminately to everyone with breasts.

Currently in Ireland the advice is that the benefits of breast screening outweigh the drawbacks if:

- you are female and aged between fifty and sixty-nine (BreastCheck should call you in every two years)
- you have a strong family history of breast cancer (in which case you may be advised to start your mammograms at an earlier age and get screened more often)
- you have been diagnosed with a gene mutation that significantly raises your lifetime risk of breast cancer (again, you may be advised to start your mammograms at an earlier age and get screened more often).

Some ladies find a mammogram quite an ordeal and are not comfortable being topless or with having a stranger manipulating their breasts. And it is true that the pressure of the two plates pressing together on to the breasts is sore. I was referred into BreastCheck a bit early – when I was forty-seven years old – because I had a painful dense area of tissue in the upper-left part of one breast where I'd had mastitis while breastfeeding. Luckily, I am not shy about having a stranger squish and squeeze my boobs on to a plastic plate and I do not find the pressure that uncomfortable (I'm not such a brave soldier, though – I need sedation to go to the dentist!). The staff in St Vincent's Hospital BreastCheck are extremely friendly and efficient, and for me the procedure is a minor discomfort for a great deal of reassurance. But I sympathize with people who dread going for a mammogram.

My advice is: go for your scheduled mammograms. I know the system is not perfect. I acknowledge all the criticisms of over-diagnosis, and the knock-on effect of over-treatment, but until a better way of diagnosing breast cancer comes along, it's all we have. And mammograms are an essential part of care for at-risk people. You should also try to be breast aware – that is, feel your breast tissue regularly, when you wash and when you are dressing/undressing. Any asymmetry or lumps or changes should be discussed with your GP.

Using HRT after you have been diagnosed with breast cancer

There have been no large-scale, reliable studies where people with different types of breast cancer were enrolled according to their cancer type and then offered either body-identical oestrogen plus a natural progesterone, or a placebo. This is how science gathers Grade A medical information. The belief in medical circles is that a study like that would never get approval. In the absence of a good clinical study, it is unlikely we will ever have a guideline to say, *If you have had this breast cancer, of this cell type and this stage and this grade, you can use this HRT but not that HRT*. Well, not in my working lifetime anyway. So, all I can tell you is what we do know for sure.

HRT is not a carcinogen. There is no direct evidence that HRT transforms healthy breast cells into malignant cells, *but* HRT hormones may have a stimulatory effect on pre-existing quiescent, pre-cancerous tumours. Or they may not. It is poorly understood. We do know it takes at least ten years for breast cells to change from the pre-malignant state to being a clinically detectable cancer. We also know that malignant changes, once they have occurred, cannot be reversed by stopping hormones. Therefore, in the absence of good studies and desperately needed information, the general approach to HRT use after a diagnosis of breast cancer has to be one of caution.

It is generally not recommended that a person use oestrogen or progestagen after a diagnosis of breast cancer. It makes total sense to be wary of HRT if you have a cancer that might grow faster or come back after treatment when you use HRT, and it is completely acceptable that, in general, doctors will usually say no to prescribing any form of HRT for a person with a breast cancer diagnosis.

But, as we know, there are breast cancers and breast cancers. Some are harder to beat than others and may shorten your life significantly. Some are survivable but may require you to have surgery, radiation, chemotherapy and hormone therapies that reduce your quality of life and may themselves shorten your life span and increase your risk of diseases such as osteoporosis and cardiovascular disease. Some breast cancers would never have come to your attention at all but for the mammogram, yet they will still be treated as a cancer and subject you to surgery or other treatments that might affect your quality of life.

Should we say no to HRT in every one of these cases?

The answer is complex. Although the overriding answer will be: *try all other non-HRT strategies.*

I regularly see experts recommend weight loss as a means to reduce flushes, like that's so easy for a middle-aged woman who has been battling obesity her entire life to just whip some weight loss out of her back pocket. (Do I sound a little triggered? Hell, yes!) But it does help, as can all the other lifestyle and non-HRT medical therapies we offer for mood changes, flushes, sweats, et cetera (outlined in Chapter 8).

It is also common to hear from patients who have been diagnosed with breast cancer and are aware of all the risks associated with HRT but would like to be involved in their own decision making. Maybe they know the risk but are still willing to venture into the unknown. They will find very little support in getting a prescription for HRT. This is in part due to the fact that, in Ireland, doctors are highly vulnerable to medico-legal litigation. If a doctor prescribes against the guidelines, they better have a darn good reason for doing so and be able to show lots of literature to support this action. If not, we might find ourselves on the stand in a courtroom, or in front of the Irish Medical Council.

You cannot expect your GP or consultant to ignore the lack of quality information and guidelines and prescribe HRT for you after breast cancer because *you* are happy to take it. It does not work like that. I have had patients demand that I prescribe HRT for them and who have offered to sign a waiver, declaring that I am not responsible if their cancer returns. In court, this sort of document wouldn't be worth the paper it was printed on, so please do not get angry with your doctors when they refuse. I understand the frustration, but the doctors are trying to 'do no harm' (as per the apocryphal Hippocratic Oath). I know of patients who booked menopause consultations with a new doctor, did not mention their history of breast cancer, and started on HRT out of sheer desperation. That is a nightmare scenario, where you are bearing all the worry and stress of managing your menopause symptoms with a doctor who knows only half the story.

The British Menopause Society is guarded in its recommendations, as you would expect. The BMS mentions the individualization of care when discussing breast cancer and HRT. It published a detailed guideline on managing menopause symptoms after a diagnosis of breast cancer. The main suggestions include the following.

- Patients should be referred to a health-care professional with expertise in gynecological endocrinology for counselling about the possible consequences of their breast cancer treatment.
- Ideally, people diagnosed and treated for breast cancer should be encouraged to try non-HRT remedies (as per Chapter 8). Many women in our Complex Menopause Service in the National Maternity Hospital have found some relief from symptoms with the use of non-HRT products, including CBT, SSRI/SNRI meds, oxybutynin and gabapentin.
- If these are ineffective, systemic hormone replacement therapy or low-dose topical (applied into the vagina) oestrogen may be considered, but only after taking specialist advice, i.e. from an oncologist or menopause expert.
- Switching breast cancer hormone treatments or taking a break from them might also be suitable, but this needs to be discussed with your oncologist.

This means that if, after exploring alternative menopause therapies, you are still experiencing a significant reduction in your quality of life and you are aware of the potential risk and have discussed the situation with your oncology team, systemic HRT might be offered *but as a last resort*.

This advice is not a great deal of help to a patient with breast cancer, or to the doctors who are trying to help them, but it does leave the door open – well, not so much open as slightly ajar – for talking about HRT as a potential treatment.

There is also the problem of variations in advice from different menopause specialists and different oncologists. I have written to many oncologists asking for help when I meet a breast cancer patient with severe menopause issues, and I can tell you that attitudes differ widely. This is very difficult for you, the patient, who is trying to learn all this stuff and make good decisions. There's a lot of work to be done to inform and support health-care practitioners, to give them the know-ledge and confidence to be comfortable assessing all options with their patients. I think it would be worth trying to get an Ireland-wide con-sensus so that, as menopause specialists and oncologists, we are on the same page in terms of attitudes to hormones and quality of life, and the other consequences of breast cancer therapies. We are working on this at the moment.

On a more positive note, there is some good news. A new style of medication is due for release soon that promises to target only those oestrogen receptors involved with flushes and sweats, while avoiding the oestrogen receptors in breast tissue (I already mentioned this in Chapter 8). These are known as the Neurokinin-3-receptor (NK3R) antagonist medications, and we hope to have them in Ireland in the near future. The plan is that they will be licensed for use in people with a history of breast cancer, so fingers crossed.

I am also hoping for an improvement in care after breast cancer diagnosis as more and more hospital-based menopause services are developed in Ireland. I expect we will collectively try to offer prac-tical but safe options for people who have had breast cancer and who are struggling with menopause symptoms.

What about using local vaginal oestrogen after breast cancer?

Vaginal oestrogen, which is considered very safe for use after breast cancer diagnosis, can sometimes provoke a negative attitude from some health-care providers. I guess it's because those products still all say *do not use if you have had breast cancer* on the leaflets – despite lots of data to support their safety. I've already discussed this at length (see pages 52–4 and 135–6).

Pelvic floor and vaginal changes are a very common side effect of breast cancer therapies. Local vaginal oestrogen is generally regarded as safe, regardless of breast cancer receptor status.

We know that a tiny amount of oestrogen gets absorbed from the vagina and into the blood when using some types of vaginal hormone therapy. The numbers are so small they cannot usually be measured by conventional laboratory techniques. A woman who has been diagnosed with an oestrogen receptor + breast cancer needs to know this because we have to ask: will using vaginal oestrogen increase her future risk of cancer recurrence or her survival?

The answer is, we don't think so – but we cannot say for certain.

Now, if you are taking Tamoxifen, the tiny increase in oestrogen level is unlikely to be an issue for you because the oestrogen receptors in your breast tissue are full of the Tamoxifen and thus protected from the effects of any extra oestrogen in the blood.

However, if you are on an aromatase inhibitor (AI), you do not have that extra layer of protection, and there may be a concern. We just can't say for certain. The limited information we do have comes mainly from a small, badly controlled UK study in 2006 and a very recently published observational study from Denmark. These studies are important and raise serious questions but are not high quality enough to provide definitive answers.

This means there is always room for discussion with your menopause or cancer specialist. The BMS suggests that if you have had breast cancer and you need GSM help, as many women do, try non-hormonal vaginal therapies first and then, if you are interested, you can use local vaginal oestrogen if **you are NOT on an AI**.

If **you ARE on an AI** and you really need GSM help, it might be worth discussing changing over to Tamoxifen – if your oncology team agrees – so that you can use vaginal oestrogen and not have this worry hanging over you.

If you have had a breast cancer diagnosis, and you have symptoms of oestrogen deprivation affecting your vagina, vulva, bladder, you should be able to use local vaginal oestrogen if you choose – particularly if over-the-counter products have not helped matters – and this is regardless of what type, stage or grade of disease you had. This is also the guidance from the UK's National Institute for Health and Care Excellence (NICE) and the menopause societies but, sadly, I still meet resistance from some medical colleagues.

Where there is a family
history of breast cancer

Most breast cancers are not hereditary – they occur randomly. A minority – between 5 and 15 per cent – of all breast cancers detected are connected to an inherited genetic mutation. The most common and best-known gene mutations that can put you at a higher risk of breast cancer are the BReast CAncer mutations – BRCA1 and BRCA2 – though there are many others that might also increase your risk.

Not everybody needs to be screened for genetic cancers. If a patient has two or more close relatives with breast cancer (and sometimes womb/ovary cancer too), we might suspect she has a cancer gene mutation running through her family. If you or a relative have been diagnosed with one of these types of cancer – especially at a young age – the oncology team might refer you to a medical geneticist. They will discuss the pros and cons of being tested.

The screening is by means of a simple blood test. You can qualify for free genetic testing if you have a certain number of risk factors. In order to be eligible, you would need to talk to your GP and ask to be referred to a screening service. There are rigid criteria for eligibility. Going for gene testing privately, to one of the services advertised online, costs about €1,000, which is a lot of money. And it can be an emotional and legal minefield, so you need to think carefully before you proceed.

Considerations on cancer gene testing

- Private testing is expensive, and the results may not be one hundred per cent accurate.
- You may find that *knowing* you have a cancer gene causes you more anxiety than the not knowing did.
- You may find confirming a cancer gene diagnosis has financial implications – for example, on health insurance and mortgage protection fees.

- Then there is the decision around telling people – are you going to share your diagnosis with your family? Will that have implications for them?

If it turns out that you do carry one of the forms of gene mutation we know to be linked to cancer risk, you might then be asked to discuss this with your family. This can be a harrowing experience for some. I think I would be grateful to get the heads-up from a sister or a cousin, so I could get tested myself and be vigilant, but I'm well aware this might not be the case for everyone.

In late April 2022, I did a talk for the Marie Keating Foundation's BRCA group. There were men and women there from all over Ireland, with lots of breast cancer doctors and medical geneticists in the audience and speaking. My sister and mom happened to be there, too, as they were visiting from the USA, and my sister was in tears listening to the stories of often young women being shamed and scapegoated when they tried to tell their family about their gene status. Who knows how anyone will feel when faced with this? It's impossible to predict.

And on top of the psychological hit, I did not know, until other speakers mentioned it, that having a diagnosed genetic cancer mutation can affect your insurance options. The nerve! That should be protected by law.

On the positive side, being diagnosed with a gene mutation that greatly elevates your risk of a certain cancer could save your life. For instance, people with the BRCA mutation will be screened often and early, and sometimes offered risk-reducing surgery that can greatly diminish the possibility of them getting breast or ovarian cancer.

Getting a handle on what having a risky gene mutation means

Women with gene mutations for breast cancer are at much higher lifetime risk of breast and ovarian cancer. Regarding BRCA1 these are the stats.

- Of 100 women in the general population, 12 or 13 of them will develop breast cancer before the age of 80. That is called background lifetime risk.

- Of 100 women with a BRCA1 mutation, 65–79 of them will develop breast cancer before the age of 80.
- Of 100 women in the general population, fewer than 2 of them will develop ovarian cancer before the age of 80.
- Of 100 women with a BRCA1 mutation, 36–53 of them will develop ovarian cancer before the age of 80.

And the numbers for BRCA2 are as follows.

- Again, background lifetime risk: of 100 women in the general population, 12–13 of them will develop breast cancer before the age of 80.
- Of 100 women with a BRCA2 mutation, 61–77 of them will develop breast cancer before the age of 80.
- Of 100 women in the general population, fewer than 2 of them will develop ovarian cancer before the age of 80.
- Of 100 women with a BRCA2 mutation, 11–25 of them will develop ovarian cancer before the age of 80.

The ovarian cancer figures are a killer as we have no early detection tools for this cancer yet.

The general advice is that if you are unlucky enough to have these genes, you already have a higher than average risk of breast cancer. You should ideally be getting regular physical breast exams and mammograms or being reviewed by a familial breast cancer service. You might even be advised to have a preventative mastectomy or oophorectomy at some stage.

Taking HRT when there's a family history of breast cancer

A family history of breast cancer can increase your own risk of getting diagnosed with breast cancer. The use of HRT on top of this appears not to *increase* risk. Long-term observational studies have reported *no extra risk* for those using HRT, or using HRT following risk-reduction surgery. HRT in such women should use minimal progestagen and ideally micronized progesterone. Recent data have shown this approach is less likely to result in a breast cancer diagnosis. If you need HRT, you can use it.

Of course, it is unlikely to be as simple as that for you trying to figure this out. You will really need to explore your own feelings towards carrying a higher than average risk of a cancer, especially breast cancer, which can be such a frightening situation for many of us. If a person who carries a known cancer gene mutation uses HRT, gets a good response, but goes on to develop breast cancer, how will they feel? Will they say, 'Damn, this was always a possibility,' and accept their lot stoically as the HRT is stopped and breast cancer therapies instituted? Or will they be filled with anger and self-recrimination, wondering if their outcomes would have been different if they had not used HRT?

There is a lot to unpick around the high risk of breast cancer and the decision to use HRT during perimenopause. Your GP is probably not a psychotherapist, and you may need someone to help you work through your own attitudes and ideas around your individual needs. If this affects you, there's good advice and discussion on the Marie Keating Foundation website and also on the Royal Marsden Hospital website – they both have excellent BRCA pages.

For someone with a known breast cancer gene mutation who has made the decision to have preventative surgery (to have their breasts and/or ovaries removed) the choice is a bit easier, I think. In the absence of breast/ovary tissue, the use of HRT is less anxiety-provoking as your risk of getting cancer is much lower – almost, but not quite, zero. That is a big decision, though, and it needs to be teased out in consultation with the oncology or familial breast cancer team, and maybe your family, too. Have a look at some of the services available for people with a cancer diagnosis, such as ARC Cancer Support Centres, a not-for-profit Irish group that offers counselling and therapies to people with cancer and their family members (www.arccancer support.ie).

The psychological toll is important to be aware of for everyone concerned: the patient, the supporter of a person with breast cancer, and the doctor trying to provide care. I learned this the hard way. The saddest stories are the worst to recall, but they teach us something, too.

I knew a lovely woman with a recent history of breast cancer. She flew through the mastectomy and had immediate reconstruction. She endured the radiation and the chemo and the adjuvant therapy stoically. She came to talk about her menopause symptoms, many of which were brought on by the cancer treatment. When she mentioned those issues to the oncologists, they said, 'Go talk to your GP.' Well, I had some options for her all those years ago, but not so many as we have now – and none of them was HRT, of course – but I felt things were ticking over, and she seemed okay. She made lots of appointments just to 'check in' – which people who pay for visits rarely do.

One day she popped in to let us know that she had been discharged by the oncologists and was only due to see them yearly from now on. She felt she had graduated breast cancer and was relieved, and we congratulated her. We got word of her suicide the following week.

I feel I could have done more. I should have been more alert to all the unnecessary visits – perhaps they were a cry for help? She did not come across as depressed to me on those visits, but of course she must have been – who wouldn't be? Surely everyone with a serious diagnosis could do with some talking therapy and other dedicated support. I think of her often and wish I had done more.

KEY TAKEAWAYS

- Some breast cancer treatments can bring on menopause symptoms, but having had breast cancer limits your choices when it comes to some treatment options. Discuss this with your oncology team before you choose a treatment pathway, and have a plan in place.
- HRT is not allowed in most cases, but there are many non-HRT options that can bring relief from symptoms, and all are worth a try.
- Vaginal oestrogen is almost always acceptable.
- A family history of breast cancer is not a contraindication to trying HRT, nor is being a BRCA gene mutation carrier, particularly if you have not had breast cancer and have had risk-reducing surgery.

19. Your bones and the menopause

Yep, the menopause goes bone-deep – taking us to osteoporosis.

Osteoporosis is a disease of the bones where they become fragile and are more easily fractured. It is linked to many factors, but a big one is declining levels of oestrogen, as happens when we go through our menopause. Without an adequate supply of our friend oestrogen, our bones start to suffer. It's important to do all you can to protect your bones throughout your life because you can end up paying a heavy price for bone deterioration as you age. But the good news is that there's lots you can do, and there's lots of medical help available to protect and treat your bones as well.

There are no early symptoms of osteoporosis, and the disease often does not become obvious until a fracture occurs – and even then it can still go undiagnosed. I bet the stats will shock you: more women die from complications of osteoporotic fractures (hip and spine mainly) than from ovarian, uterine and cervical cancers combined; fewer than 15 per cent of osteoporosis sufferers are ever diagnosed, according to the Irish Osteoporosis Society; approximately 50 per cent of women and 20 per cent of men will experience an osteoporosis-related fracture in their lifetimes; the burden of disability from osteoporosis on the health services is greater than for all sites of cancer, with the exception of lung cancers. By the way, by 'fracture' doctors have in mind cracks in the bone as well as broken bones. (There is also a pre-osteoporosis condition called osteopenia – see page 227 for explanation.)

The complexity of your bones

Our bones are a complex organ structure that truly knows how to multi-task. Their jobs include:

- holding us upright and supporting all our muscles so that we can stand and move
- protecting our soft, squishy bits from injury
- helping to balance the mineral content of our cells and blood (bone contains almost all of our body's calcium and phosphate and about half of our magnesium)
- playing a key role in the formation of new blood cells – these are formed in soft tissue inside our bones (the bone marrow)
- acting as a storage facility for our triglycerides – these are stored deep in the marrow.

The outer, shiny white part of bone is called compact or cortical bone and it makes up 80 per cent of the total bone volume. Bone is extremely strong. Cortical bone has holes and channels running through it that carry blood vessels and nerves. It is the cortical bone that holds us upright and gives our muscles, ligaments and tendons somewhere to anchor.

Inside this outer layer of bone is the other 20 per cent of bone, which is known as spongy, trabecular or cancellous bone. As the name implies, it's spongier in nature. It's made up of a network of tiny pieces of bone arranged in a twisting, convoluted lattice structure – like a honeycomb (imagine the inside of a Crunchie bar). This part of the bone gives us some flexibility so that when we jump or fall, our strong, outer cortical bone doesn't just shatter. Cancellous bone has lots of spaces in between the latticework and that is where our bone marrow is found.

When we are babies and young children our bones are soft and bendy and actively growing – this is because they do not have much mineral content in them yet. Then as we enter puberty, our hormones help control the rate at which the body starts to lay down calcium and other minerals in the bone, giving it much more strength. Puberty hormones also close off the ends of our long bones (so we don't keep growing taller and taller for our whole lives).

In females, the main puberty hormone is, of course, oestrogen and it helps to control bone strengthening and maintenance, and allows us to achieve what they call our peak bone mass, which is our maximum potential bone size and strength.

Lots of factors help decide what anyone's peak bone mass will be – our genes are among the main players there – but other things can also influence the development of our peak bone mass, things like lifestyle factors, poor diet and minimal or excessive exercise, and excessive alcohol intake. Hormones, too, play a big role in laying down bone and bone minerals: the healthier the levels of oestrogen you have as a teenage girl and young woman, the better your ultimate peak bone mass can be. Similarly, lack of oestrogen will prevent you achieving your peak bone mass. Men usually achieve a higher peak bone mass than women because men lay down more bone than women, and their bones are wider and bigger anyway. Women have smaller bones, so that makes us a little more likely to experience osteoporosis as we age.

Men and women usually reach their peak bone mass by their mid-twenties or around thirty years of age. By the time we reach the age of forty, we are all – even really healthy people – slowly losing bone. But some people start to lose it too quickly. Although everyone will lose bone with age, people who have achieved a higher peak bone mass when young are better protected against the natural drop in bone mass that comes with aging.

How osteoporosis develops

There are cells in bone that are in charge of wear and tear and general maintenance. These are the *osteoclasts*. They melt away and dig out damaged bone, leaving a gap. Then the *osteoblasts* lay down new, fresh bone to fill the gaps. This process of bone digging up and bone laying down is called *coupling*. Without oestrogen – say, in menopause or in POI – the osteoclasts lose the run of themselves and dig out more bone than the osteoblasts can keep up with. This results in bone loss.

Think of it like bone roadworks. There are two separate crews – lads who dig the holes and other lads who fill them in – only the hole-digging lads are super-fast and the hole-filling lads are very slow. If you tell the Department of Bone Roadworks to take on more jobs, there will be loads and loads of holes because the slower team can't catch up with the work. The decline in oestrogen speeds up the coup-ling process, leaving the hole-filling lads far behind in their attempt to catch up with the hole-digging lads. Osteoclasts require weeks to melt bone, whereas osteoblasts need months to make new bone. So, any process that increases the rate of bone remodelling or coupling – like the loss of oestrogen in menopause – results in net bone loss over time, and this bone loss is *osteoporosis*.

A silent disease – diagnosing osteoporosis

Osteoporosis is a largely silent disease until a fracture occurs, and even then it often goes undiagnosed or untreated because some doctors forget to consider osteoporosis as a cause of your fracture. If you break (fracture) a bone as a result of a simple slip or fall (as opposed to being hit by a truck, say), you need a DEXA scan. Fractures as a result of minor accidents are known as 'fragility fractures' or 'low impact fractures' – meaning a person with healthier bones would most likely not have ended up with a broken bone after a similar incident – but you did, so something is up. The only way to diagnose osteoporosis is by getting this DEXA scan, which may show that your bone density has dropped below what we think is a critical level.

One thing that I'd like to reassure you on is that aches and pains in the joints are *not* a symptom of osteoporosis. I often have women in the clinic who ask for a DEXA scan because they have joint pain and it is seriously worrying them. I have to explain each time that one does not mean the other. And it doesn't.

What is a DEXA scan?

A DEXA scan is a specialized bone X-ray that measures your bone mineral density (BMD) and compares the density of your bone to the ideal bone density, which is characterized as that of a healthy 29-year-old person of the same sex as you. (They use a 29-year-old as the base because that's the age at which bone density reaches its maximum potential. It starts falling thereafter.) The difference between your bone density and the 'ideal' bone density is called the T-score. Another result you can get from a DEXA is called a Z-score, which compares your bone density to that of other people of your own sex and age.

If you have a T-score of 1, your density is 'ideal' – that is, it is the same as a healthy 29-year-old of the same sex as you. If you have a T-score of −1, your bone density has dropped one standard deviation below ideal. This score doesn't indicate a disease – it just lets you know something's going on. Things get serious when your T-score drops below −2.5. When that occurs, you are diagnosed with osteoporosis, and you need to be treated for it.

Osteopenia – a sign that you are losing bone mass

Before you hit osteoporosis, there's an intermediate stage that might be identified on your DEXA scan. If your T-score is −2.4 you are not one hundred per cent safe from osteoporotic fractures, but you don't officially have osteoporosis yet either. Bone specialists call this osteopenia, a weird middle area where your bone density is low, i.e. worse than −1 but not worse than −2.5. Loads of people have fractures with osteopenia, though. In fact, according to statistics from the Irish Osteoporosis Society, most people who experience a fracture are found to be in the normal and osteopenic density ranges: 50 per cent of fractures occur in osteopenic people, 40 per cent in osteoporotic people and 10 per cent in people whose bone density is considered in the normal range. Therefore, the goal of diagnosis is to identify people who are at risk of either fragility fracture and/or osteoporosis as these two situations are not the same. When assessing your risk of osteoporosis, your doctor should take a full history to see if you have any factors that put you into a higher risk category for fracture – for example, if there's a history of osteoporosis in your family. Some basic bloods might help too, such as full blood count, liver function tests, thyroid hormone levels, vitamin D and calcium.

Lots of people with osteopenia will get a broken bone, but treatments are usually based on finding out why your T-score is dropping and fixing that, or offering therapy to help slow down and maybe reverse this drop. By the way, the word osteopenia means 'less bone'. It was a term coined in 1992 at an osteoporosis convention. A group of World Health Organization (WHO) bone metabolism experts (rheumatologists) were cooped up in a hot and sticky Roman hotel room for days, trying to decide where the T-score number should be to make a diagnosis of osteoporosis. Some felt −2.5 was too low and that osteoporosis should be diagnosed with less bone loss. Out of desperation they agreed on the −2.5 threshold but suggested that doctors also keep an eye on anyone at −1 or lower. They decided to call those people 'osteopenic'. So, osteopenia isn't officially a disease, like osteoporosis; it's a heads-up that you are losing bone and that you need to do something to slow down the process.

How do you know if you are at risk of a fragility fracture?

You can assess yourself using either FRAX or QFracture® algorithms. These are websites where you input your details and they calculate your risk of having a broken hip or other major bone fracture in the next ten years – a pretty neat diagnostic tool that can be extremely useful in forward planning and treatment options.

FRAX is the Fracture Risk Assessment Tool, developed in 2008 by the WHO Collaborating Centre for Metabolic Bone Disease at Sheffield University in the UK. It calculates your ten-year probability of a major osteoporotic fracture and hip fracture using a computer-generated algorithm. It is the most widely used fracture risk assessment model in Ireland, but it has no specific validation for use in Irish people. It relies predominantly on your age and DEXA scores, however, so it generally comes into use when you are already some way down the path of diagnosis and treatment.

By contrast, QFracture® doesn't rely on a DEXA X-ray score for its accuracy and extends to populations ranging from thirty to eighty-four years of age. FRAX might be more suitable for people aged between forty and ninety.

For patients who are curious about their bone health but not seemingly at very high risk, I would do their FRAX assessment without a DEXA scan first and if they score healthy, then they probably do not need to rush off for a DEXA scan. However, if they get a bad FRAX score, I would definitely get them to have a DEXA scan, to get a full picture of what's going on with the bones. If they had a very high FRAX risk, I would start a treatment while waiting for the DEXA appointment, which can take weeks and weeks depending on where you live.

Why some people are more vulnerable to osteoporosis than others

There are a number of different risk factors that affect your likelihood of developing osteoporosis.

- *Age* : the older you are, the more likely you are to be diagnosed with osteoporosis, but it is not inevitable and there are some risk factors that can be managed so as to limit your own personal risk.
- *Sex* : being an older female increases your risk because the rate of bone coupling in women is directly linked to the levels of oestrogen in the blood.
- *Nutrition and physical activity* : your bones have to last you a lifetime, so it's important to eat well, exercise regularly but not obsessively, and don't smoke – all the usual advice for healthy living – to maintain good bone health.
- *Genetics* : hereditary factors play the principal role in determining an individual's peak bone strength, accounting for up to 80 per cent of the variance in peak bone mass from one person to another.
- *Hormones* : your hormones also play a big role in bone quality and the risk of osteoporosis. This is why menopause can have such a big impact on bone density because of the loss of oestrogen. After the age of sixty, men start catching up with the women as their hormones start declining, increasing their risk of osteoporosis too.
- *Ethnicity* : pale people have weaker bones than dark-skinned people. This likely relates to millennia of sun exposure. Vitamin D is important for bone health and it's formed by exposure to sunlight.

- *Thin build or small stature* : e.g. body weight under 9 stone/57 kg, low BMI exposes you to more fracture risk, as does being very tall and thin.
- *Amenorrhoea/oligomenorrhoea/late menarche/early menopause* : in each case, usually because of lack of oestrogen.
- *Physical inactivity or immobilization* : movement stimulates bone-forming cells (osteoblasts) to be activated, while inactivity leads to less bone formation, which can lead to osteoporosis.
- *Medication use* : e.g. anticonvulsants, systemic steroids, thyroid supplements, heparin, chemotherapeutic agents, insulin and PPIs have all been shown to affect bone density.
- *Alcohol abuse and tobacco use* : both reduce bone density.
- *Calcium deficiency* : good calcium intake is important for the maintenance of bone.

If you can count some of these risk factors in your own medical history, you should be alert to the fact that you have an elevated risk. You should discuss that with your GP and ensure you are monitored accordingly. However, it's usually the case that osteoporosis generally does not become obvious until a fracture occurs.

The most common bones to break as you age are the wrist and collarbone, hips and ankles, as well as crunch breaks in the vertebrae of the upper back. Hip fractures are usually pretty obvious when they happen, but minor cracks with minimal pain can slow down detection and treatment. But it might not be that clear cut. Two-thirds of back bone (vertebral) fractures are painless, for example, but some vertebral fractures might be accompanied by an episode of acute pain after a fall or minor trauma. We often hear of patients remaining motionless in bed for fear of causing an exacerbation of the pain. Acute pain usually resolves after four to six weeks, but multiple upper-back fractures can result in kyphosis or bent spine, otherwise known as 'dowager's hump'. (You've seen those poor older ladies bent over like a question mark – it makes me so sad to see because that is fully preventable.) Then the pain may become chronic. Signs include local tenderness over the cracked vertebra in acute cases, and a decrease in height of 2–3cm after each vertebral compression fracture. Progressive kyphosis can result from these compression fractures, which reduces your quality of life and mobility, and can affect how you breathe.

Preventing and treating osteopenia and osteoporosis

Prevention is better than cure and you may well have a sense of your own risk factors. I am built like a hobbit, I hill-walk and I'm on HRT, so my chances of getting osteoporosis are pretty low, I hope. As you can see, some of that is genetics (thanks, Mom!) and some is my lifestyle.

You can also be aware of your own risk level and adjust some of those modifiable risks with your behaviour and lifestyle choices.

- *Diet* : eat a balanced diet rich in calcium and vitamin D.
- *Exercise regularly* : increased muscle strength may prevent falls by improving confidence and coordination, as well as maintaining bone mass and preserving muscle strength. Weight-bearing exercises are best at stimulating bone growth, so try dance or Zumba or do hill-walking. A daily thirty minutes of weight-bearing exercise helps prevent bone loss.
- *Mobility* : immobilized patients may lose as much bone in a week as they would otherwise lose in a year. For this reason, immobility should, wherever possible, be avoided – even if you're laid up in hospital with a fracture or bone break.
- *Smoking* : cut down or stop! Ask for nicotine replacement – it helps.
- *Vitamin D* : supplements of 800 units daily are usually sufficient. If you're at risk of osteoporosis or already being treated for it, it's usually recommended to take calcium and vitamin D together for a healthy double whammy.
- *Calcium* : supplements are inexpensive and may increase BMD up to 1 per cent over two years. Post-menopausal women need 1–1.5g calcium daily. Ideally, you should get your calcium by eating calcium-rich foods, like dairy products, bread, tinned fish and green vegetables. But if you decide to

add in a supplement, just make sure to take into account how much you're already getting from your diet and also check the concentration of calcium in the supplement (the percentage of *elemental* calcium). It is actually dangerous *not* to be on calcium if you are also on a bone drug, as the bone drug will be pulling calcium out of your blood and getting it into your bones to fill in the holes. Too little calcium in the blood can cause heart problems – take the calcium tablets if you are on bone drugs, please.

- *Fall prevention*: correction of decreased visual acuity, reducing consumption of medications that alter alertness and balance, and improving the home environment (slippery floors, obstacles, insufficient lighting, handrails, small pets – that last one's from painful personal experience!) are important measures aimed at preventing falls.

There are plenty of medicines that can help to stop further bone density loss and reduce your risk of fracture, and also medicines that can actually help you to build back lost bone. The choice of which medicine to put you on depends on how bad your condition is and what you can tolerate.

If you are at high risk of osteoporosis, or you have had a fracture or broken bone, there's a very good chance your treatment can be managed by your GP to start with and then maybe get some help from our colleagues on rheumatology. In fact, you do not always have to get a DEXA X-ray and a T-score before commencing treatment, particularly if your fracture risk is considered to be very high (but we will get you that DEXA scan to assess your exact bone status as soon as possible).

There are circumstances with osteoporosis when you'll need more help than your GP can provide. When this is the case, you can be referred to secondary care in the form of rheumatology outpatients or, in some cases, a falls clinic. A referral might be in order where:

- the osteoporosis is unexpectedly severe or has unusual features at the time of initial assessment
- the patient has complex medical conditions known to be associated with osteoporosis

- there is intolerance of therapies or the patient is experiencing problems
- the patient sustains a fracture in spite of treatment or normal bone density
- the GP does not have access to DEXA scans.

HRT and other treatments for bone health

Prior to the WHI study publication in 2002, HRT was considered the gold standard for both prevention and treatment of osteoporosis for women in menopause. As many women then feared breast cancer from HRT use, other osteoporosis treatments were used.

Now that we understand the shortcomings of the WHI study, HRT is back on the table as both a treatment and a preventative therapy for osteoporosis. Several menopause societies as well as the UK's Royal Osteoporosis Society have published a Position Statement on *The Use of HRT in the Prevention and Treatment of Osteoporosis*. This says that:

> HRT is an effective treatment for menopausal symptoms and offers protection against fractures at both hips and spine. For women affected by osteoporosis aged under 60, HRT has a role to play in the management of osteoporosis.

For women under sixty who are at high risk of osteoporosis and who want HRT, it should be a first-line option. After the age of sixty, we need to weigh up the risks and benefits more carefully, so we would probably not start someone who is over sixty on HRT just for bone health – unless they had menopause symptoms or some additional reason to use HRT. Where that doesn't apply, we would probably go for a bone sparing medicine, like a bisphosphonate, or the antibody denosumab.

Bisphosphonates are anti-osteoclast drugs. Remember, osteo-clasts are the super-fast hole-digging lads in our bone roadworks crew, so these drugs are used to slow them down, to help improve bone density and reduce fracture risk. GPs start women on bisphos-phonates all the time. Like any medication, they are not without risks and side effects – doctors have worries about their extended use as this can lead to unusual fractures later in life – so a good chat about them as well as your options/alternatives is wise before you start.

Denosumab is a six-monthly bone density injection that can be offered by your GP. It both slows down osteoclasts and speeds up osteoblasts (the lads filling in the holes), giving excellent protection from osteoporosis and reducing fracture risk. Unfortunately, new data have emerged showing that once you start this denosumab drug, your bones become dependent on it and if you stop, the osteoporosis comes back with a vengeance, so no easy solution here either.

It is imperative that women with early menopause or POI are on some form of HRT, if at all possible, as they are at a greater risk of osteoporosis, having started the low oestrogen phase of their lives so young. They should be recommended to start HRT and encouraged to continue their HRT until at least the normal age of the menopause (fifty-one), in order to reduce bone loss – as well as to improve menopause symptoms.

The diagnosis or fear of osteoporosis often helps to encourage women who are unsure about trying HRT because they know that, as long as they are on the HRT, their bones will be stronger all the time. Women under sixty who use HRT for menopause symptom relief can be reassured that the benefits of HRT will exceed the risks, and that the potential bone protective effect will be an additional benefit. If at any stage they choose to stop the HRT – as most women usually do – they may need to consider some other osteoporosis-preventing or reversing drug.

If you can't take oestrogen, which will apply to women who have had certain types of breast cancer, or would prefer not to, the usual advice is to work on good lifestyle habits and perhaps take either denosumab injections or a bisphosphonate tablet once the BMD starts to drop below −2.5 or if you have already had a fragility fracture, but this needs to be teased out with a rheumatologist.

In case your doctor mentions them to you, here are some other medications and treatments that might be suggested, depending on the state of your bone health.

- Selective oestrogen receptor modulators (SERMs), such as raloxifene or bazedoxifene. These are not as powerful as standard HRT for fighting osteoporosis, but they are considered safer for people who have had breast cancer.
- The dual action bone agent strontium ranelate can be used in severe circumstances. This is only offered by rheumatologists and only if you are already badly osteoporotic.
- Teriparatide (parathyroid hormone) – again, this is for severe cases.
- Surgery – hip replacement, vertebroplasty and kyphoplasty are all awful operations you do not want if you can avoid them. So, if you are at high risk for osteoporosis, I encourage you to read this chapter again; you'll find lots of ideas in it to work on maintaining your bone health, starting today. And get in to talk to your GP!

KEY TAKEAWAYS

- ☒ Osteoporosis is an often-silent bone disease that can be prevented if you are on the lookout for it.
- ☒ Lots of things you do or don't do contribute to your osteoporosis risk – fix them where you can.
- ☒ HRT will prevent and treat osteoporosis in eligible women, but it only works while you are taking it.
- ☒ There are many osteoporosis treatments that do not involve HRT if you do not want it or have been told not to use it.

PART IV

Menopause and particular health issues

20. Endometriosis – walking the tightrope when it comes to menopause care

Endometriosis is a common chronic inflammatory disease of the reproductive system, and people with a history of endometriosis have to be a little bit more careful when it comes to exploring their options for menopause care and HRT.

Endometriosis describes the disease when the cells and tissue typically found only in the lining of the womb (the endometrium) start to grow in other parts of the body. It becomes a problem because normal womb-lining is designed to thicken, shed and discharge out through your vagina. If endometrial tissue grows in other places, not just in the uterus, it still does its thing every month: gets thick, undergoes cellular changes and gets ready to bleed and shed. And if that tissue can't get out of the body, it will stay trapped inside, causing pain and inflammation, with lots of potential for complications. The most common parts of the body where you might find errant womb-lining tissue can include:

- inside the muscles of the womb (aka adenomyosis)
- on the walls of the pelvis
- in/on the fallopian tubes
- on the ovaries
- on the bladder or in the walls of the bladder
- on the surface of the bowel
- near or on your pelvic diaphragm
- in your caesarean section scar(s).

In some crazy cases, you can find endometrium in very distant sites, such as the lungs. I remember reading a case where a girl had endometrium tissue at the back of her eye, in her retina. Every time she had a period, she bled through her tear ducts, like in a religious apparition. I've never actually seen a patient like that, though. The most common symptoms I see in general practice are varying degrees of cyclical, pelvic, maybe menstrual-type pain to start with. The strangest case I personally treated was a woman with endometrium tissue on her diaphragm, which was causing monthly chest pain. Why this strange migration of womb-lining tissue occurs, no one knows for sure – theories include, among others, an inherited gene and backward-flowing menstrual tissue.

Apart from a lot of pain, the trapped tissues can cause internal bleeding and scarring, or adhesions can form. Adhesions are a thick band of springy tissue – they look a little bit like those balls of elastic bands made by bored office workers – and they can stretch from one part of your insides to another, trapping tissue and organs inside this unhealthy network of scar tissue bands. Trapped bits of organs and tissue can cause lots of pain and eventually might cause you to develop other complications, if not treated (for example, loops of bowel, or other structures, getting tangled up in adhesions, which can cause acute pain and trips to the Emergency Department). Fertility may be affected if the endometriosis involves your ovaries, your fallopian tubes or womb muscle.

The big problem with endometriosis and its symptoms is that it can be a relatively silent affliction; meaning the degree of pain you *feel* may not reflect the severity or the extent of the endometriosis. Not only can endometriosis cause varying amounts of pain and other symptoms, it is incurable – that is, we can *manage* it, but we can't get rid of it entirely. It is a true medical nightmare for some people.

The pain of endometriosis can be considerable and can be triggered when you exercise or try to have sex, when you have a bowel motion or have a pee. You can even bleed into your bladder and find that your urine turns pink, or there might be some blood in the poo when you have a bowel motion. Sometimes the pain becomes permanent and persistent, and in many cases it has a profound and distressing negative impact on quality of life. So many people grit their teeth and put up with it, never really speaking about what they're going through. The loss of well-being, loss of productivity in school or in work, the effect on your social life and life choices is hard to measure, but it is thought to be enormous. Endometriosis is one of the most common causes of low fertility, occurring in between 30 and 50 per cent of women attending fertility clinics. Reactive depression (a non-clinical depression brought on by stress or distressing circumstances) is associated with all sorts of chronic medical conditions, but it is a very common complication of endometriosis.

The challenge of diagnosing endometriosis

Endometriosis can be tricky to diagnose without directly looking inside your pelvis, which is why many people go undiagnosed and untreated for years, if not forever. The main symptom is pelvic pain, but unhelpfully this doesn't always hit around period time. Of course, period pain is terrifically common – not just in people with endometriosis. And if you complain of pain associated with periods, there's a chance you'll be told that periods are painful and so, more or less, just *suck it up*. But people who may have found that their period pain was manageable when they were in their teens can find themselves feeling much worse pain in their twenties and thirties – and they could have endometriosis.

The gold standard test to diagnose endometriosis is a laparoscopy – or looking into the pelvis with a camera while you are asleep. This clearly shows any endometrial tissue that's hanging out where it doesn't belong, and then a sample of the tissue (biopsy) can be taken and sent to the lab for confirmation of the diagnosis.

Unfortunately, we can't perform a laparoscopy on everyone who complains of period/womb pain. That's simply because this kind of pain is very common, so you'd quickly have a list that went on for years if you started sending everyone for a laparoscopy – and the slots would be filled up with people who really were having bad menstrual pain but no actual endometriosis. On top of that, a laparoscopy involves a general anaesthetic, which has risks attached including, on rare occasions, death. Then there is the cost to health care – with limited budgets in public hospitals, every laparoscopy operation for suspected endometriosis means another operation you're not doing for someone else. Lastly, because we can treat you for endometriosis without necessarily knowing for certain that you have it, everyone with period pain does not and should not have a laparoscopy. The guidelines for mild endometriosis that has not affected your fertility are: assume you might have it, treat it and only send for full work-up if things are not improving – and that is what your GP will often do. This is known as 'empirical treatment'* and we are urged by guidelines to do this in general practice all the time.

This means that going to a gynaecologist and having a laparoscopy is usually not necessary when your GP has a good working knowledge of endometriosis guidelines and care. However, a laparoscopic evaluation is much more important if:

- empirical treatments aren't working
- you're showing signs of the complications of endometriosis, such as acute episodic pain (for instance, a cyst on your ovary might rupture and you could end up in the ED thinking your appendix is exploding – it's serious and it can be dangerous)
- you are trying to conceive and find there is a delay in getting pregnant.

In those cases, you definitely do need to see a gynaecologist and have more advanced care.

GPs need to know all about endometriosis because it is a fairly common condition, with around 20 to 50 per cent of women with infertility having some degree of endometriosis and around 30 to 80 per cent of women with pelvic pain having it. Officially, around 10 per cent of females in Ireland are living with the diagnosis, but this is likely an underestimation as so many sufferers won't get as far as a proper medical diagnosis.

If you have a suspicion that you might have endometriosis, you need a GP who knows their way around women's health issues. To do so, I would recommend checking out practice websites – if they have a website, that's a good first sign. If they specifically mention women's health on their website, even better. If you get an appointment, email

---

* Empirical therapy is when we choose a treatment based on experience and logic rather than a definitive diagnosis. In medicine, we always remind ourselves that common diseases are common and consider them first before referring you for high-tech, possibly unnecessary investigations. If you do not respond to empirical treatments, then you definitely need further tests. Let's try this and see, basically.

in advance to say you need someone with experience around gynae issues and see what response you get. Alternatively, you could choose to attend at your nearest Family Planning Clinic or Well Woman Centre.

Periods are unnatural!

My perspective on period pain, and on endometriosis and its treatment is this: while a certain amount of cramping and period pain is natural and to be expected for all people who menstruate, *it is not necessary*. There can be a little bit of an old girls' club attitude towards periods sometimes, like, *I got through it without medical help, why can't you?* Or, *That's just the way it is for us girls.* I call BS on that: it doesn't make you less of a person if you choose not to be doubled over on a couch for hours/days at a time due to this 'natural' process we call a period. There is no value in going through this monthly 'rite of passage' and, indeed, it is neither unhealthy nor unnatural to shut that shit down and get on with your day like other people do!

Here's why I think periods are unnatural: the female mammal is made for making babies. Young humans with wombs are typically fertile from puberty and are physically designed to make babies and have healthy pregnancies. Every month you get a chance to use one of your limited supply of eggs to get pregnant. We used to do this soon after our periods started as a young teen, basically because there was no way to stop it happening and because, with shorter life spans, getting pregnant young and often was a good thing. Now, that doesn't suit most of us any more because we want to live our younger lives without the responsibility of being a mother, so that we can pursue an education and get some living done – and rightly so. But every month when you do not get pregnant, you are arguably putting yourself in an *unnatural* situation, i.e. shedding an egg and having a period.

It might sound odd to modern ears, but women weren't designed to have periods that frequently. Take a hundred years ago, women often had twenty pregnancies from sixteen to forty-six years of age, with about ten or fewer periods in between because they were always either pregnant or breastfeeding. We were like puppy mills! That took its toll physically, of course, but on the flip side you never heard much about endometriosis back in those bad old days. (Of course, no one would have listened if those ladies did mention pain, but that's for another book.) Things like womb-lining cancer and ovarian cancer were rare too, because these are often diseases linked to women with no/few pregnancies. But this is the twenty-first century and teens in the developed world usually avoid pregnancy – and that's fabulous, I believe – except that this can lead to a few gynaecological problems, with endometriosis being a big one. It's a side effect of the freedom we enjoy – a bit of a kicker from good old Mother Nature.

We know that a pregnancy can cause endometriosis tissue to shrink and disappear. Simulating pregnancy can help fool the body. So, if you have bad periods, if you lose time out of your period week due to heavy flow or pain, get help. When we use relatively safe and healthy medicines to simulate pregnancy, block wasted ovulations and turn off that rotten period, that is not 'unnatural'. It is actually trying to return your body to the more natural state of not ovulating all the time (i.e. not 'wasting' eggs every month) and may in fact improve your health and even your fertility.

The main treatments for endometriosis

There are plenty of different treatments available – and new therapies, such as selective progesterone receptor modulators, are currently being developed – so ask for some options before you decide. Look through the treatments below as a starting point. Remember, though, that there is no cure for endometriosis, no way to treat it that guarantees it won't return. If you use a treatment, you must stay on it long term. You can't start and then stop when you feel better. This is a mistake I see people making all the time. *Oh I went on the pill for a year and felt better, so I came off it.* Ah no – you do not know the rules!

Painkillers

Painkillers, especially anti-inflammatory painkillers, can help to control the cramps and will reduce, to a certain degree, some of the internal inflammation that contributes to endometriosis pain. Anti-inflammatory painkillers include Ponstan, which is the trade name of mefenamic acid, which is regularly prescribed for period-related pain, aka dysmenorrhoea. Ibuprofen is another well-known and regularly used one, although not everyone can take it – some people react to it badly.

Physiotherapy

Alongside pain interventions, physiotherapy can be a big help. There are wonderful pelvic floor physios in Ireland who should be involved in a multi-disciplinary approach to endometriosis. You can access a physio privately – check online for information, and look for a pelvic floor physio service – and you can also get referred to a hospital-based public service by your GP.

Anti-ovulation contraceptives

The combined hormonal pills, patch or ring all act to shut down brain signals to the ovary that commence ovulation. If you don't ovulate, you don't get so much womb-lining growth, which results in less bleeding/less pain/less damage from endometriosis. Other contraceptives that shut down ovulation and can really help with endometriosis include the mini-pill or progestagen-only pill (POP), the Implanon-NXT implant and Depo-Provera injections. Even a Mirena coil, which does not usually shut down ovulation, can help with some types of endometriosis, particularly where there is tissue growing in the womb muscle. Again, these contraceptives will only help while you are on them, so you must stay on them – whether you are at risk of pregnancy or not – as coming off them will allow your endometriosis to kick off again.

GnRH analogues

These are a class of high-tech medicines that can only be prescribed by a specialist. They cause a chemical menopause in your brain and block the development of endometriosis. These are the heavy-duty weapons, and can bring on loads of side effects, therefore they must only be used under careful supervision.

Surgery

Surgery to remove some of that endometrial tissue and the adhesions can be carried out at the time of the diagnostic laparoscopy operation. This is not a straightforward fix, however, as the burning/cutting of the surgery can result in its own scar tissue and adhesion formation. For that reason, this is not undertaken lightly and is usually reserved for people who did not find medications effective or who are battling infertility. In terms of surgical solutions, as a last resort you might be recommended to have your ovaries removed, to stop ovulations once and for all. Or, if things are very bleak, you might be advised to have surgery to remove either the womb, the tubes or anything else that may be matted down with endometriosis scarring and adhesions. But this is a very serious situation that we hope to avoid by early and ongoing intervention with some of those other, simpler therapies.

The relationship between endometriosis and menopause/HRT

The normal cells of the womb-lining are under the influence of the famous four cycle hormones: oestrogen and progestagen, FSH and LH. The oestrogen causes womb-lining thickening, while the progestagen affects the cells of that lining. During the second two weeks of a monthly cycle, progestagen levels climb in the hopes that you have conceived. The elevated progestagen hormone nurtures the womb-lining to promote the possibility of a healthy pregnancy. When it becomes obvious to the body that you did not get pregnant, progestagen levels drop and this results in womb-lining release, i.e. your period, and the cycle starts again.

As you get older and your ovarian hormone levels fluctuate and then drop, endometriosis *usually* improves because there's less hormone feeding its development. (Now, this is too simple an explanation, of course, as there are some well-documented cases of endometriosis only showing up *after* the final menstrual period.) For most endometriosis sufferers, though, the final menstrual period should bring an improvement to the degree of discomfort and pain they have been experiencing and also to the consequences of endometriosis.

Obviously, if you reverse that hormone loss by adding in external hormones, as we do through HRT, that could easily have an impact on the course of endometriosis, so that has to be taken into account.

Some people have had their menopause thrust upon them overnight by endometriosis treatments, like GnRH injections or oophorectomy/hysterectomy, and for these ladies there is a great need for oestrogen replacement. But if we add in even the gentle oestrogen of transdermal HRT, we might stimulate the remaining endometriosis tissue, and back to square one they go.

Caring for women with menopause symptoms and a known diagnosis of endometriosis is a nuanced business. When we add back some oestrogen to replace or balance the hormones to tackle menopause symptoms, we need to also try to suppress the remaining endometriosis tissue. We usually do this by offering progestagens. We do this even when there is no womb. If you have had your womb removed and you want HRT but you had moderate to severe endometriosis in the past, you should probably use progestagen along with your oestrogen (even though you don't officially 'need' the progestagen as you have no womb-lining). You still ought to take it because it should help suppress a flare in the old endometriosis tissue.

The progestagen should be offered in a daily regime because using it cyclically (2 weeks on/2 weeks off) will just drop the suppression of the endometriosis tissue and lead to problems. After a few years of daily oestrogen and progestagen, you may be able to get away with oestrogen-only HRT after your hysterectomy as your endometriosis tissue may well have regressed on its own. We can't be doing monthly laparoscopies on people with endometriosis when they are on HRT, so we are usually led by their reports of pain and other symptoms and strive to get the balance right. Even so, we may need to get help from our gynae colleagues to make sure everything you need is being taken into account.

KEY TAKEAWAYS

- ☒ Endometriosis is a common and often under-diagnosed condition.
- ☒ It may improve when your natural periods stop, so using HRT may cause it to flare up again.
- ☒ Using HRT is not contraindicated in women with known endometriosis, but it does need careful prescribing and monitoring.

21. Menopause care for transgender people

The information you've been reading throughout this book applies to anyone who was born with a womb and ovaries. We all share a common experience when it comes to hormones, menstruation and menopause, even though it's obviously very subjective and there are many stories within those experiences. But for those people born with a womb who later choose to live as a man — whether they choose surgery or not, hormone treatment or not — the experience comes with some additional layers that can make it more challenging. I want to acknowledge the transgender population directly here and give you any information that's available and that might apply specifically to you.

That said, I'll start with a frank admission: there isn't all that much specific information available because the necessary clinical studies have not yet been conducted. I'll just straight up confess that this won't be a long chapter, and that I have limited information to hand, but I'd still like to address this topic directly, as much to raise badly needed awareness as anything else.

When knowledge and medical experience are lagging behind your lived experience, that's really hard on the transgender person because there's always that justified fear that you won't be well received or, if you are, that you won't get the help you need. So, it's important that we medics recognize that the transgender experience of peri-menopause and menopause is real, and often complicated, and requires specialist information and training.

I'm going to explain transgender from a medical point of view, using the terms currently used in the profession. Some of this may seem a bit 'Transgenderism 101' for those in the know, but the purpose here is to raise awareness and knowledge among those who don't know, to give some insights into the experience, as well as to give information to transgender readers, so bear with me while I set out the stall nice and clearly. And might I also acknowledge that the rest of the book uses the terms 'women' and 'men', 'female' and 'male', which may have been difficult for some transgender readers. I apologize if that's the case for you.

What do we mean by transgender?

Transgender (TG) or gender diverse people are a small but growing group in Ireland. A cis★ person is born with sex organs, and their gender identity matches those sex organs. Therefore, a cis woman has female genitalia and feels like a woman, or a cis man has male sex organs and feels like a man. A transgender person is born with sex organs that do not match their sense of gender identity or sense of self. A transgender woman is born with male sex organs but identifies as a woman. Likewise, a transgender man is born with female sex organs but identifies as a man. In other words, they do not identify with their birth-assigned sex or their 'biological' sex.

A gender identity mismatch may create a personal conflict for someone because their outward ('obvious') gender presentation may not sync with how they feel about themselves or how they want to be perceived in the community. This is why the treatment and surgery that 'correct' physical gender characteristics in a gender diverse person are called gender-affirming treatments or gender-affirming surgeries, because they *affirm* the correct gender for that person, regardless of the physical attributes they were born with.

There can be many variations of TG identity and, as you may start to guess, I am no expert in this area, just a clumsy ally doing my best. But it is important for the TG community that we accept and understand their needs.

This really hit home for me recently when I met a TG man who was on a contraceptive injection to shut off his periods but was experiencing unusual vaginal bleeding. When I walked into the waiting

---

★ Cis comes from the Latin, meaning 'on the same side as'. Trans means 'across' or 'beyond' or 'on the other side of'.

room, my heart immediately went out to him. Just imagine sitting in a gynae clinic waiting room, the only person not obviously female, not a hundred per cent sure how you will be received and treated. I escorted him into the consultation room, introduced myself and explained what my role was (basic clinical skills) and then asked what his preferred pronouns were before we got things under way. He was so surprised, he couldn't speak for a moment. When he confirmed that 'he/him' were the correct pronouns, I could hear the emotion under his answer. He told me that not a single medical person – doctor or nurse – had ever asked him that question before. That broke my heart.

It was the first time I truly understood just how important this is for the TG man or woman. It means everything to them to be respected for who they are – not who you think they should be. By asking that simple question and hearing the answer, it immediately creates a safe space where they can talk openly and trust that they will receive appropriate and respectful care. And this is a note for my colleagues: it is on us – the medical practitioners – to create those spaces, and it takes so little to do it. How does a non-cis person convey that to you before they reach the surgery? We need to look at practical things, like registration forms – are there only two boxes to tick, male or female? This has practical implications because how can a GP do an automatic referral for a TG woman for prostate screening if she is automatically registered to the practice as female? It just takes a bit of planning and sensitivity. Be kind and gentle and open – as you should be with all patients – as the person before you might be rattling with nerves about this encounter.

The transgender experience of menopause

If you are trans, there are multiple factors to consider, such as your chromosomal make-up, the sex organs you had at birth and whether they are still present or not, the medications you are being prescribed (and are actually taking), or other hormone therapies you are using and intend to use. For example, if you are on hormone blockers, you need supplemental hormone therapy as use of hormone blockers alone can expose you to long-term risk with regard to bone density and

liver function, among other things. It is usual for people on blockers
to be advised to take hormone supplements, too, so as to balance this
risk. Health care for transgender people, including menopause care,
requires a comprehensive discussion with a trusted doctor to build up
your personal bigger picture, taking into account your own risk factors and how you can tackle them, and also, if you choose, some help
with reducing menstrual bleeding.

For transgender men

If you have the sex organs that were present at your birth (ovaries,
womb, cervix, vagina, et cetera), then throughout your life you will
need to maintain them with interventions like cervical screening, and
possibly you will require help with reducing menstrual bleeding. You
may also require contraception, and that will need to be aligned with
your hormone therapy, be it for menopause or otherwise. You may
also want to consider freezing eggs or embryos prior to hormone therapy or surgery, just to leave that door open for later consideration.

In later life, if your birth sex organs are present and you have not
taken oestrogen blockers, you will start perimenopause and enter
menopause. If you had an oophorectomy (removal of ovaries), that
means you've already gone through surgical menopause – and hopefully you will be using male hormone therapy to replace the lost
oestrogen. You will no doubt have been advised, stemming from that
surgery, to stay on your testosterone supplements – usually for life.
If this is the case, the good news is that you are unlikely to experience the typical ovarian hormone decline that cis women go through
in mid-life. Nonetheless, you need to be breast aware – even after a
mastectomy – and you should be familiar with your normal chest tissues and, ideally, should attend BreastCheck for regular screening after
the age of fifty if you have not had a mastectomy.

For transgender women

If you have the sex organs that were present at your birth (penis,
testicles) and have not used oestrogen, you won't experience perimenopause or menopause. Ideally, you should regularly self-examine the

scrotum if you still have testicles, and be aware of any signs of disease, like pain and swelling. Even if you have had your testicles removed (orchidectomy), you need to attend for regular prostate cancer screening. It is true that female hormone therapy reduces prostate cancer risk, but screening is still wise and advisable as it will monitor for benign disease as well. If you have been on oestrogen, you need to be aware of your breast cancer risk. Regular breast self-examination is essential and you can also sign up for regular screening via the BreastCheck programme.

If you had an orchidectomy and have been taking oestrogen hormone, you may have been told to consider stopping that oestrogen at the age of fifty, or you may decide yourself to stop using hormones as you get older. If you do choose to stop, this may cause problems for you. We know cis women can suffer when their natural oestrogen levels become unpredictable and then decline – and this will almost certainly be an issue for you coming off your oestrogen therapy.

The amounts of oestrogen prescribed for transgender women are usually higher than the amounts used in the menopause care of cis women because we are, of course, not only supporting your fluctuating hormones but also supporting your gender transition. The maximum dose advised for transgender women is 6mg of oral estradiol daily (or 150mcg in a patch, gel or spray), which is much higher than the most common dose of HRT oestrogen (2mg oral or 50mcg in a patch, gel or spray). If you are on combined hormonal contraception products or oral oestrogens, that will increase your risk of thrombosis, so you will need to optimize other risk factors, like overweight and smoking. As I've said many times already in this book, mid-life can be a watershed for all of us – cis and trans – so it is time to embrace common-sense lifestyle choices that can help you age in as healthy a way as possible.

You may have been on female hormone therapy for many decades, and we do not have an abundance of data on how this may affect your current or future health. We know cis women with POI may be on similar amounts of oestrogen until the age of fifty, at a minimum (and, in their case, often progestagen and low-dose testosterone as well). Guidelines for POI care tell us to keep those younger women on the hormone therapy until at least the average age of menopause. They are advised to talk to their prescriber about when/if to reduce the dosage or whether to come off it altogether at that point. It follows that a discussion about whether or not to stop taking oestrogen and/or trying a lower dose or changing to a better delivery system (transdermal versus oral oestrogen) is also wise for you as a TG woman when approaching your fiftieth birthday.

Getting menopause and mid-life health care as a transgender individual

You probably don't need me to tell you that we are a long way from the perfect Irish health service – especially when it comes to gender diverse people. What you will be hoping to find is a health-care provider who is open-minded and willing to self-educate on LGBTQ+ information and can therefore provide a safe space for your menopause discussion. Sadly, this is not as simple as it should be.

On the medical side, education about transgender issues for health-care providers, be they doctors, nurses, pharmacists or physiotherapists, is not mandatory nor is it standardized. Some of us may get quite a good understanding of transgender health issues during our undergraduate or postgraduate training, but some of us hear very little indeed. I certainly had no core training in gender diversity, and I never met a transgender or non-cis patient during my training – not that I knew of, at any rate.

While there are online resources for interested GPs, viewing them is not mandated in any way, so there can be a wide range in terms of knowledge and reaction from one doctor to another when you seek health care. I'm writing this in autumn 2022, and that's how it is right now, so all I can do is be honest about that and hope it changes quickly.

Of course, some doctors will have loved ones or friends who are transgender, and therefore will have self-educated in an effort to support the person they love. But it's really a hit-and-miss affair, which is very tough on the patients looking for our help.

There is work being done in this area now, to bring this issue into the light and make sure health-care professionals are aware of it and engage with it. In the February 2021 review by the Irish College of

General Practitioners (ICGP), for example, there was a clear reminder of how important health care is for gender diverse people. It stipulated that all health-care professionals must be 'open, non-judgemental, understanding and supportive'. I hope that is the experience of gender diverse patients, but I apologize on behalf of the profession if this is not your experience.

As new generations of doctors, nurses and other trans-aware and trans-supportive professionals qualify and start working in the health service, trans people should be more confident of meeting know-ledgeable and non-judgemental health-care professionals. For the time being, however, you have to negotiate the medical landscape as it stands.

Depending on your situation, there's a good chance you might not experience symptoms of perimenopause. However, if you do need to access care and support around menopause, look for GP practices that list menopause as an area they specifically cover – that's a good first step. I know some wonderful GPs who are themselves members and/or supporters of the LGBTQ+ community and could be a good fit for you. There is no index or anything like that, so the best advice I have is to Google *LGBTQ* and *family doctor* and *Ireland* and see who pops up. I found some excellent doctors that way.

If you are nervous about describing your medical history to date, or if you don't feel able to recite it chapter and verse each time you meet a doctor or nurse, you could try drawing up a bullet-point list to cover all the key information. This way, you can either email it to your GP in advance or let them read it when you arrive for your consultation, then you take the discussion from there, rather than you having to take a breath and do a deep dive into your personal history. The reaction you get to that document will tell you a lot about the doctor, which should be helpful in choosing the right person to work with you on figuring out the best menopause approach for you.

KEY TAKEAWAYS

- ✍ Medical colleagues who work closely with TG patients often remark that many of their patients simply stop taking their meds of their own accord, and don't return to the clinic. I would encourage all TG people facing menopause to find a doctor they can talk to, and to keep up regular visits and reviews. It might not be in your best interest to stop all medication at a certain age – it would be preferable to make that decision together with an informed medical professional.

- ✍ Currently there are limited specific services for TG patients in Ireland, but there is the National Gender Service in Loughlinstown. The Complex Menopause Clinic at Holles Street accepts transgender patients for menopause consultation and care. You need to try to find a good medical partner to help you out over these years.

- ✍ A key takeaway for my medical colleagues: it's up to us to be knowledgeable about the needs of our TG patients and to create a safe space for them in our clinics.

- ✍ If you are seeking information on all matters relating to TG people, including medical issues, a good resource is www.teni. ie, the website of Transgender Equality Network Ireland.

22. Living with excess body weight and the menopause

Before I dive into this, I have a reading recommendation. *Fat Is A Feminist Issue* is a landmark book by British psychotherapist Susie Orbach. The title says it all. It's forty-five years since it was published and it remains relevant to this day. It covers the whole shebang of us and our bodies – how we women see ourselves, the societal and internal struggles many of us have around body image and size, our self-worth, and its relationship to our bodies . . . I could go on forever. In this chapter, however, I am going to conveniently ignore all that and just discuss body weight and its possible impact on our physical health.

Measuring body weight

In medical terms, you are classed as 'overweight' when your body mass index (BMI) is greater than 25. The formula is to divide your weight in kilos by the square of your height in metres. The result tells you if you're 'underweight' for your height (under 18.5), 'normal' (18.5 to 24.9), 'overweight' (25.0 to 29.9) or 'obese' (30 or greater). Don't try this at home – just find an online BMI calculator and they'll do the sums for you!

If your BMI gets to 40 or over, that's classed as severely obese. Being obese means that your weight has become a medical condition in and of itself, and it is likely going to have a significant negative impact on your health.

Now, while BMI is crude, and therefore somewhat controversial – for instance, a big strapping muscular rugby player might come out as overweight or obese simply because there's no way of tweaking the formula to allow for his big build and shedload of muscle – it has some use as a medical tool, as long as we don't jump to conclusions and we properly probe people's health story with them, taking *all* factors into account. The BMI index makes it seem like a simple, cut-and-dried series of markers, but in reality, there's so much involved in each individual case.

A new perspective on excess body weight

When you've attended at a GP or clinic as an overweight or obese person, there have probably been times when you felt that the doctors and nurses blamed you for your weight, that you felt they were thinking, *Jeez, if only you could just eat less and exercise more, you wouldn't be carrying all that unnecessary weight. You'd have a healthier life. And all would be well.* That attitude has been a problem, let's be honest, and it's an extremely simplistic and not particularly helpful point of view. While the 'eat healthy/exercise more' advice might be a solution for some, many people already do those things and continue to have a high BMI.

Nowadays, we health providers are starting to look at obesity and being overweight in a different way. There is growing understanding that overweight/obesity can be a chronic medical condition – in much the same way as having headaches or being diabetic is – and that, as with any other chronic medical condition, the person needs compassion and support, not judgement and a 'tsk-tsk' attitude. Some people do not metabolize the food they eat in the same way as others. Even if they eat well and exercise, they retain ingested calories as stored fat rather than burning them off. For many of these people, the only way they would ever be able to keep their BMI under 30 is to live a spartan lifestyle of severe calorie restriction, which in itself could have a negative impact on their quality of life.

Some people are just hungrier than others. The areas of the gastro-intestinal tract, liver, pancreas, fat cells, et cetera, as well as certain areas of the brain that control satiety, such as the brain stem, the cortex and the hippocampus – those areas that help you feel full – might not be working at optimum levels in some people. There are hunger hormones that get released when you are thinking about eating, when you start to eat, and others that kick in when you are full. Your ability to feel full after you've eaten is as much a part of you as your eye colour – and it can be changed to help you manage your weight.

Obesity is a global pandemic of its own, with most of the developed world affected by it. In the USA, around 66 per cent of adult Americans are overweight; in Ireland, 60 per cent of adults and 20 per cent of children are overweight. In response, medications for appetite and weight control are constantly being developed by pharmaceutical companies, albeit with minimal success. Some of the earliest products were a form of methamphetamine, which was associated with a fair few side effects, not least of which were psychological and physical addiction. About twenty years ago, we saw the release of fat blockers that could reduce how much fat you absorbed from the foods you ate. These medicines can help – but if you're not *extremely* careful about the amount of fat you eat, you can end up with a highly fatty content to your bowel motion and experience stomach cramps and explosive diarrhoea. So, not an easy solution there either.

Over the last twenty-five to thirty years, surgical options have been explored. Bypassing the stomach, or putting a band around it to reduce its capacity, not only cuts down on the amount of food people are able to eat, but also affects the hunger centres in the brain and the hormones that control appetite. Many people have achieved dramatic weight loss after banding or bypass procedures. However, most clinics no longer recommend banding as the complication rate is too high and these people frequently go on to need bypass anyway.

Therefore, gastric bypass surgery or bariatric surgery (i.e. surgery relating to the treatment of obesity) are currently the preferred surgical options to help manage obesity and to cure non-insulin dependent (type 2) diabetes. These are popular surgeries and highly recommended for people living with severe obesity whose medical health is affected to a significant extent. When you remove certain parts of the stomach, long before you lose a single pound in weight, your type 2 diabetes goes away. It's complex, but changes in the pancreatic cells involved in producing the blood sugar-reducing hormones insulin and amylin are seen immediately after the operation, and secretion of glucagon-like peptide-1 (GLP-1) – a gut hormone that reduces appetite – is increased. It's basically a miracle to me, and I'm sure it feels that way to people who have been struggling with their diabetes.

Bariatric surgery is not an easy option, though. It is not available to all in Ireland and even if you are eligible, the waiting lists are long. Some people are tempted to access cheaper surgeries in other countries, where the risks of the surgery and complications afterwards are very high. To be blunt, you could die – so please do not get a low-cost flight to a weight-loss place until you've tried all the medical strategies available for weight loss through your GP or other health provider. Also, while gastric bypass operations are miraculous for diabetes, they may not always be a permanent solution for people living with obesity because the stomach can stretch, hunger levels can go up again, and the weight can pile back on.

So, what are the other medical strategies you can try? Medicines that affect those hunger and insulin centres have been developed over the last decade or so – drugs that mimic the effect of GLP-1. Bariatric researchers discovered that after your gastric bypass operation, the small bowel begins to produce different hormones, some of which help the body to use glucose. Working on from this, scientists have developed ways of synthesizing medications that have a similar biochemical impact on diabetes as having a gastric bypass – without the need for surgery! As a result, injectable medicines are now available that reduce glucose levels in people with diabetes (type 2) but also, amazingly, help reduce appetite and control weight. We now know that these meds can be used safely by obese people who are not diabetic. In spring 2022 a licence was granted for a drug known as semaglutide (a GLP-1 analogue) to be offered to obese people for weight control. This is good news for those who need help with their weight, but there are still some hurdles.

- First, many GLP-1-type meds are taken by self-injection, which would put a lot of people off – although an oral version of semaglutide has just been licensed and should be available in Ireland soon (after mid-2022).
- Second, these drugs cost big money and they not covered by the Medical Card or Drugs Payment schemes unless you have diabetes, in which case you can get them on the Long-Term Illness (LTI) Scheme.
- Third, sometimes you might be tempted to stop them, and this would be counterproductive.

I struggle with my weight and I have tried an injection version of semaglutide (trade name Victoza) and it really helped, but I did miss eating and being starving and tucking into a lovely big dinner. The weight didn't fall off or anything like that, but my appetite was reduced. Although I can get a bit hypoglycaemic at times, especially when I'm hill-walking, so now I bring a big bag of Maoam sweets with me, just in case. Actually, that is a lie, my hiking buddies bring the sweets as I always forget and they are fed up listening to me whinge about feeling 'hypo' on the hills! As with lots of things, motivation is a big factor. But it is good to know that if weight is an issue for you, and it's affecting your quality of life, there are non-surgical medical interventions that can help, and more and better options are coming on stream regularly.

Menopause and weight gain

Menopause is associated with weight gain – what the heck isn't, I hear you cry! But yes, for a lot of women as they age and their oestrogen levels falter and eventually drop, their metabolism is affected. You might find you are eating the same foods and taking the same amounts of exercise, but your weight starts to climb anyway. When it comes to menopause, this weight gain is the result of a hormonal shift. The drop in oestrogen levels can affect where fat gets deposited, so instead of a bigger backside and hips, which is known as gluteo-femoral weight gain, you get more belly fat and more central body fat. This deposits the fat near your important organs, which is more closely linked to disease risk. Cardiovascular disease risk is especially increased both by central obesity and falling oestrogen levels.

So, on top of everything else, menopause can make keeping your weight in check even more challenging. Unfortunately, HRT does not directly make you lose weight and might even make you feel a bit puffy/bloated when you first try it, as some people retain fluid when they start out on a sex hormone medicine. Any fluid retention or bloating from the progestagen component of your HRT will typically settle and improve after two to three months. If you start HRT and you feel your bras don't fit right, or your trousers won't close, it is possible that this will settle naturally over the course of three or four months as your body gets used to the new steady level of hormone. If it doesn't, or if these symptoms are particularly severe and you just can't cope with them, go back to your prescriber and together you can consider trying a different brand or a different cocktail, maybe a lower dose hormone, maybe a different delivery system, maybe a different progestagen.

While saying that HRT won't make you lose weight, on the other hand if you weren't sleeping, if you were exhausted and finding it hard to exercise, if you were turning to crappy foods because you needed some comfort while going through your difficult menopause time, then on all those counts HRT may help you to keep your weight down. It's possible that getting yourself some good menopause treatment will give you back a certain amount of quality of life and let you approach exercising, weight control, et cetera in a better frame of mind.

Many patients living with excess weight and obesity ask me if it's safe for them to be on HRT. I think confusion often arises when we think of the hormones in the contraceptive pill, which are also oestrogen and progestagen, in contrast to the hormones in HRT. We would never give the combined oestrogen and progestagen contraceptive pill to someone who was living with significant obesity, especially if they were also over thirty-five years of age. It would be even more critical to avoid the oestrogen + progestagen contraceptive hormones if that person also smoked or suffered from migraines. This is because we know that the high-dose artificial oestrogen found in the pill, patch and ring – mainly ethinylestradiol – is linked to a higher risk of blood clots, as is being overweight, as is smoking. So, occasionally, when a HRT-prescribing doctor meets an overweight or obese person seeking help with menopause symptoms, they worry about whether or not it would be safe to give them HRT because they remember the caution surrounding the combined contraceptive pill hormones.

For total clarity: *HRT is not the pill*. HRT is totally different. The rules about prescribing HRT are completely different from the rules about the pill. The hormones in HRT are much less powerful and we tend to use them in more modest doses, too.

In addition, as a person living with obesity goes through the menopause, her risk of weight-related diseases, especially hypertension, cardiovascular disease and diabetes, starts to climb. By balancing and replacing the oestrogen in her blood and tissues – especially the low-dose, non-oral, no clot risk HRT oestrogen in the gels, patches and spray – we can actually help protect her from CVD, improve her sugar balance and reduce her systolic blood pressure. So, not only is it safe to go on HRT if you are living with excess weight or obesity, it may even reduce your risk of CVD and diabetes and hypertension.

Crucially, you and your GP need to be selective with your products. Generally, we would avoid oral oestrogen in HRT for people who are living with excess weight or obesity and defer towards the non-oral, transdermal oestrogen products. This is because we know low-dose transdermal oestrogen, as found in HRT, has a neutral impact on blood clot risk. Even a woman who had a blood clot while on the pill or when pregnant could use HRT, although in that case a chat with a menopause specialist would be advisable. And in terms of progestagens in HRT, certain high-dose artificial progestagens have been linked to blood clots, but again this just means that you need to be aware of this and make a careful and judicious choice of progestagen when selecting your HRT combination if you are overweight or obese.

KEY TAKEAWAYS

- ☒ Overweight/obesity is a chronic disease and needs thoughtful, modern advice and interventions.
- ☒ Menopause hormonal changes can make overweight/obesity even worse, but HRT may help slow that down.
- ☒ While the contraceptive pill may not be safe in some overweight/obese people, transdermal HRT is safe and can be safely prescribed.

23. Managing your menopause with diabetes

Diabetes mellitus literally means 'honey pee' and it refers to a medical condition whereby your body cannot efficiently process the glucose in the food you eat and drink. Instead of being able to burn that glucose for energy in your cells, it gets trapped in your blood and then lost into your urine. You may end up feeling tired and thirsty all the time, you may find that you get more infections or gain weight too easily: these are telltale signs of diabetes. Left uncorrected, the extra sugar in your blood can lead to damage in your skin and organs. It is a serious medical condition at any stage of life.

The two main types of diabetes

Diabetes is on the rise and, according to Diabetes Ireland, there are approximately 266,000 people living daily with diabetes today, and this is expected to increase to 280,000 by 2030.

There are two main types of diabetes.

- *Type 1 insulin-dependent diabetes mellitus (T1DM)* is an auto-immune disease in which the body's own immune system attacks the insulin-producing cells in the pancreas. Insulin is the hormone that helps your body use sugar for energy. If you have no insulin, you have no sugar-processing control.
- *Type 2 non-insulin-dependent diabetes mellitus (T2DM)* may be acquired over time as a result of your cells becoming resistant to insulin, or you not having enough insulin to deal with the amount of sugar and carbohydrates you consume; 90 per cent of people with diabetes have this kind.

One of the potential triggers for diabetes is menopause. Oestrogen has an effect on insulin production and release, as well as on the sensitivity of your tissues to insulin, so menopause, and the sudden drop in oestrogen levels in your body, brings a slightly higher risk of developing type 2 diabetes. And if you already have type 2 diabetes, the perimenopausal hormone fluctuations, and then decline, aren't going to do your diabetes any favours either.

So, can you take HRT to manage menopause symptoms if you are diabetic?

Yes, you can – but you have to be extra careful. HRT has a beneficial effect on sugar balance, even in women who do not have type 2 diabetes. Now, HRT is not, of course, a substitute for diabetes meds, weight management, exercise, smoking cessation, et cetera – all of which are key for women who have type 2 diabetes – but it won't do you any harm either. HRT may even help you feel better, sleep better, which in turn will help motivate you to do all the hard work that comes with being diagnosed with type 2 diabetes.

Type 1 diabetes is a risk factor for osteoporosis, so in addition to symptom relief, HRT may be of benefit in osteoporosis treatment and prevention, too.

Diabetes is not a contraindication to HRT, but we would typically choose a non-oral oestrogen and one of the quality progestagens for patients who have type 1 or type 2 diabetes. The main reason for this is to avoid the small additional impact that oral oestrogen adds to blood clot risk, given that people with diabetes are slightly more at risk of venous thromboembolism (see next chapter).

People with diabetes are also at a higher risk of heart disease, so avoiding the oral route for oestrogen helps there, too. We need to deliver your oestrogen in the gentlest way possible.

Women with diabetes are at a slightly higher risk of womb-lining cancer, too, so using a quality progestagen in good doses and investigating any unexplained bleeding is really important. When I say 'good doses', I mean the correct dose. Women with diabetes can sometimes bleed too much on the standard progestagen doses in HRT, so it's important that their doctor takes that into account and finds the correct dose. We might need to bump up your progestagen dose, for example – and we would be quicker to scan that womb-lining if it starts to bleed unexpectedly.

KEY TAKEAWAYS

- ☑ Diabetes is an important chronic disease that, left uncontrolled, can lead to lots of serious health consequences.
- ☑ It can flare up or develop around the time of menopause.
- ☑ HRT use is not contraindicated in women with diabetes – either type 1 or type 2 – and may benefit sugar control, but if you already have serious medical problems linked to your diabetes, it may be sensible to see a menopause specialist or talk to an endocrinologist (a specialist in diabetes) prior to trying HRT.

24. Menopause, HRT use and the risk of blood clotting

Oestrogen has a powerful impact on the chemicals that control the flow of blood in our veins and arteries. Medical people and lots of patients are aware that high levels of oestrogen in the blood is 'pro-thrombotic'. In other words, oestrogen can promote and enhance the mechanisms by which blood clots inside the blood vessels.

What is a blood clot?

When a patient talks to me about a 'blood clot', they might mean a congealed puddle of blood cells, like the kind you might see on a sanitary pad during a period. Those kinds of 'blood clots' are fairly normal and not dangerous insofar as blood that you have already bled is meant to gather into clots or clumps, if there's enough of it. Obviously, too much menstrual blood with loads of clots is a sign that your period might be too heavy for optimal health, and you might want to talk to your doctor about that, but these kinds of clots of blood are not dangerous in and of themselves.

Other times, we might describe something as a 'blood clot' when we mean the clotted areas of blood that can form under your skin when you've hurt yourself and you end up with a bruise – also not dangerous, and pretty common.

But when we say 'thrombosis', this type of blood clot is a whole different ball game. A thrombosis ('thrombi' in the plural) is a small collection of blood cells that gather *inside* your blood vessels. Clots of blood inside your arteries or, more commonly, inside your veins are dangerous, they can cause lots of damage and may even be fatal.

Many things increase your risk of developing a thrombosis in your artery or vein. Certain types of female hormone are included in that list. Thrombi can occur in any blood vessel in any part of the body, but one of the most common types is known as a *deep vein thrombosis (DVT)*. A collection of blood cells, fibrin, platelets and white blood cells can gather and progressively collect, often around the valves of the deep veins, usually in the legs or pelvis. They can block the return of blood to the heart through that vein, which may cause pain and swelling and a sensation of heat, but sometimes a DVT is silent and causes no symptoms at all.

Worse yet, a piece of a DVT can break off and travel. When this happens, it's called an embolus, i.e. a travelling thrombus, and it can end up in the veins of your lung. When you get a blocked vein in your lungs it is known as a pulmonary embolism. Deep vein thrombi can travel around the body to your heart, causing a heart attack. Or they can travel up to your brain, causing a stroke, all of which could possibly be fatal. As a group, these clots that can form in the deeper veins are often referred to as venous thrombo emboli (VTE).

Why DVT and VTE happen to some people but not to others is not always clear, but there are loads of clues and known risk factors.

The risk factors for deep vein thrombosis

Age

The older you are, the more likely you are to suffer a DVT. This is because you are more likely to develop other thrombosis-related conditions as you age. Also, your platelets seem to get stickier as you get older, which adds to your thrombosis risk.

Immobilization

If you do not move your body, the muscles do not squeeze the blood in your veins back up to your heart as efficiently, so it pools in the lower half of your body and is more prone to gather into a thrombosis. Bed rest of more than three days is linked to thrombosis, which is why people in hospital wear those tight stockings that are meant to help blood get squeezed back up to the heart. This is also why you're recommended to wear compression stockings on long-haul air flights.

Pregnancy and the postpartum period

Certain hormonal states affect blood clot risk, and pregnancy is a big one. In fact, the few weeks right after you give birth are the riskiest time of a pregnancy to get a thrombosis. Why this happens is to do with the fact that being pregnant is linked to clottier blood. We describe pregnancy as a 'prothrombotic state', in that you have the big three factors happening in your body at the same time.

- *Venous stasis*: your blood is pooling in your lower body because the pregnancy hormones reduce the tone of the muscles in your entire body, including the walls of your veins, not to mention your growing belly is pushing down on the blood vessels in your pelvis and abdomen. This effect on the return of blood to the heart lasts for about six weeks after you deliver, so keep active and follow other post-childbirth advice, please.
- *Endothelial damage*: the inside lining of the walls of your veins is stretched and damaged from the pressure of the pooled blood in them, especially the veins in your pelvis and legs.
- *Hypercoagulability*: this is the most important risk factor in pregnancy. A combination of changes in clotting factors, making your blood stickier, creates the perfect environment for a thrombosis. Some of these changes in clotting molecules are probably a good thing, so that you don't lose too much blood in delivering your baby, but the payback is hyper-sticky blood. We believe it is the high levels of oestrogen in a pregnant woman's blood that lead to this hypercoagulability.

Smoking

There is a bit of controversy here because while smoking definitely increases the risk of clots in your arteries, it is less clear if it increases vein clots, too. However, it does seem to be worse when you smoke a lot. Smoking raises the level of certain molecules in your blood, leading to your blood being more 'clottable'.

Inherited clotting disorders

Some people are born with a higher risk of thrombosis. If you have a parent or sibling who has been diagnosed with a clot and there was no obvious trigger for it, then you may have an 'inherited thrombophilia' and need to be cautious yourself.

Major surgery

For about four to six weeks after a big operation, especially a pelvic operation, and especially if that operation was for cancer, your risk of thrombosis is elevated. About 25 per cent of people who end up with a thrombosis get one after a surgery. Why is this? General anaesthetics are given with muscle relaxants, the muscle relaxants affect the width of your veins and the vein walls, which can lead to an increased risk of thrombosis. Plus, you are lying still and not pumping back blood to the heart during and after your operation. In addition, you might be laid up in bed for longer after a big pelvic operation. Some people are given anticoagulation injections before and after their surgery to prevent thrombosis, and everyone who can is encouraged to 'mobilize' after an operation.

Long plane or car journeys of more than four hours in the previous four weeks

Again, blood pools because you are sitting around for hours with your legs hanging down. (I am increasing my risk right now writing this book!) In addition, high altitude on long-haul flights causes changes to your blood oxygen, as well as the added risk of the dehydration we all seem to get on long-haul flights, and this adds to thrombosis potential. So, when on a plane, move around the cabin, wear loose clothes, and drink water. Do not get hammered and pass out in a sitting position (my dad's patented technique, God rest him) – this is not good for your veins.

Cancer

About 20 per cent of people with cancer will get a thrombosis. Cancer affects your clotting molecules, making your blood stickier. Some cancer treatments will have this effect, too. Again, being less active/ bed-bound will increase the pooling of blood in your legs and lower body.

Previous DVT

There is residual damage in a blood vessel that has already had a thrombosis, which means the damaged area attracts more clot-forming platelets. Some high-risk people get put on blood-thinning drugs for a long time after a DVT – although these medications can cause their own problems.

Lupus

Fifty per cent of people with lupus also have antibodies for fats (phospholipids) in the walls of their cells. If you have anti-phospholipids in your blood, you are more likely to develop a clot. Mind you, you can have anti-phospholipids and not have lupus. Tricky. (See Chapter 26 for more on lupus.)

Some contraceptives

Any high-dose, strong oestrogen – like the ones in all the combined pills, rings and patches – can increase thrombosis risk; similar to the elevated risk linked to being pregnant. Some progestagens have been linked to increased DVT risk too, but not at the typical doses we see in progestagen-only contraceptives, thankfully!

How do female hormones affect thrombosis risk?

Oral oestrogen goes straight from your stomach to your liver, where it is metabolized, and it is in there, in that first run through the liver, where the oestrogen affects some of the clotting molecules. This can result in a higher risk of thrombosis. We call it the 'first pass effect'. This risk is mostly elevated when you've just started the pill/patch/ring for contraception, so using them for a short time is not safer than staying on them for months or years. In fact, every time you switch brands or come off your oestrogen + progestagen pill for a few weeks or months 'to see if everything is still working in there', you increase your clot risk when you restart. (Try not to do that. If you like your pill and are happy with it, then just stay on it. You gain nothing by taking a 'little break'; unless you have decided you don't want contraception any more or you are trying an alternative method. In that case, just stop taking your contraceptive pill completely.)

We do not/should not prescribe contraceptives with oestrogen in them to people who already have an elevated risk of clotting and DVT, so if you are a smoker and you smoke a lot (more than twenty a day), you should probably avoid the pill, patch and ring. But even lighter smokers need to start thinking of getting off oestrogen-based contraceptives as they get close to the age of thirty-five because clot risk seems to climb around then.

If you are overweight, if you have lupus with those anti-phospholipid antibodies, or have a past history or a strong family history of DVT clots, we do not recommend these contraceptives. Even oestrogen contraceptives that you take in through the skin or the vagina (the patch and the ring) will affect your clotting risk because they are much more potent than natural body-identical estradiol in a HRT patch. That means the contraceptive patch and ring are no safer than the pill when it comes to clotting risk.

Does HRT oestrogen affect your risk of blood clotting?

Yes, even the oral oestrogen in HRT can increase clot risk, but there is an abundance of research to confirm that low-dose, natural HRT oestrogen – the kind that avoids that first pass around the liver after you swallow it – does not affect clot risk. This is supported by all the menopause guideline groups, as well as by the gynaecology and haematology guidance groups. So, if you use typical doses of HRT patches and gels and spray, your risk of blood clots is whatever your own background personal risk is anyway – no higher.

People who are smoking, overweight or who have had a blood clot in the past should not use oestrogen contraceptives nor should they use oral oestrogen in HRT, but they can all safely try transdermal oestrogen. According to the UK's National Institute for Health and Care Excellence (NICE):

> The risk of venous thromboembolism (VTE) is increased by use of an oral oestrogen-containing HRT product compared with baseline population risk, but the risk associated with transdermal HRT given at standard therapeutic doses is no greater than base-line population risk.

Now, here is the tricky part: *having had a clot in the past makes you higher risk for another clot in the future*. If this happens to you when you are on transdermal oestrogen HRT, you might think that the HRT made that happen. It didn't, but it is possible other medics will tell you that it did. So, a long chat with your HRT-prescribing doctor is important when people with a history of DVT want to start HRT. The British Menopause Society (BMS) recommends that if you have a personal history of DVT or VTE, you should have your first HRT assessment with a menopause specialist or a knowledgeable haema-tologist (blood clot specialist).

Here's another tricky bit: all the information leaflets that come with transdermal oestrogen – and even with vaginal oestrogen, which has never been suspected of increasing DVT risk – will say, *may cause blood clots* or, *do not use if you are at risk of blood clots*. If only we could get pharmaceutical companies – or, more precisely, their lawyers – to update their product information leaflets!

A large review of thrombosis and HRT was published a few years ago in the *British Medical Journal*. It helped us confirm what we had been observing – that is, people on non-oral oestrogen HRT might get a DVT, but their risk of this is the same as people who are not on HRT. This study did not actually review micronized progesterone, for some reason, but it did look at dydrogesterone and found it also to be a safer option when there is concern about blood clots.

KEY TAKEAWAYS

- If you have a blood-clotting disorder, you can take low-dose transdermal oestrogen, if you wish.
- If you are on warfarin (oral anticoagulant) or a NOAC (novel oral anticoagulant aka non-vitamin K oral anticoagulant) or DOAC (direct oral anticoagulant), you can also take low-dose transdermal oestrogen. You will need to check this with your medical team.
- You ideally need to talk to a menopause or blood clot specialist first, if at all possible, before you try HRT.

25. The effect of menopause and HRT on headache and migraine

Headache is a common but also quite complex medical problem. You can have simple headache, sinus headache, tension headache, cluster headache and migraine headache, among others. Some women get menstrual headache, linked to the last few days of their monthly cycle. For some, medications can cause headache. You can get a headache from a little too much wine or from a brain tumour. Because headaches are unpredictable and a very individual phenomenon, knowing your way around headaches, and their possible link to hormones, is a big part of what we do in general practice.

Some people find they only start to get regular headaches as they approach perimenopause, while others find their headaches improve around this time, and others say nothing has changed either way. HRT can have an impact on headache, too. Some people who have only recently started getting menopause-related headaches find HRT helps alleviate the problem, while others who never had a headache in their lives get their first one when they start HRT.

How HRT will affect your headache status is anybody's guess but having a history of headache is not a contraindication to HRT. Indeed, if you have found that your headaches only started or got worse during perimenopause, HRT may well give you relief. It's like throwing darts blindfolded – you hit, you miss, you're not sure what the heck is going to happen next.

Now, *migraine* is a separate topic for us as doctors. Migraine is defined as a moderate to severe headache – often causing pain on one or other side of the head, or behind one eye, and it can last for hours or days. It is usually associated with other symptoms, such as intolerance to light, nausea/vomiting and fatigue, and in many cases weird autonomic nervous system symptoms, almost like the symptoms of a mini-stroke, such as weakness in a group of muscles, loss of speech, or

visual changes that affect one part of the field of vision. These neurological features usually start – and then resolve – before the headache
comes on: they are the warning alarm sounding to tell you a headache
is in the post. This is known as a 'focal migraine' or a migraine with
an aura. Occasionally, the neurological warning signs come, but no
headache follows. This is an atypical focal migraine.

I get focal migraine myself, from time to time. These are severe
headaches that can last more than twenty-four hours. They are almost
always preceded by a kind of neurological warning sign. Typically for
me, about thirty minutes before the headache kicks in, the bottom
right-hand corner of my vision becomes altered. It's like I'm trying
to look through broken glass. If I look up to the left of my field of
vision, I can focus. But if I look down and to the right, all I see are
broken, bright lights. I always start by rubbing my eyes and thinking to
myself – did I look straight into a light bulb? That's what it feels like.

This visual aura is very common in migraine sufferers. It is known
as a 'scintillating scotoma', which sounds prettier than it feels, I can
tell you. But I have learned to recognize this warning sign and act on
it. If I take my favourite migraine medicine with a chaser of a large
dose of paracetamol, I can often get away without developing the
headache at all – and possibly even go on to do my work and have my
normal day's activities. But if I don't get the headache medication in
before the aura resolves/before the headache starts, I'm going to be
floored for the next twenty-four hours, minimum. (I can only use
rectal medication for the headache, by the way, because I also start
throwing up, too – such fun!)

When I was pregnant for the third time, I got an aura whereby my
right hand wouldn't move when I wanted it to. I kept dropping the
cups I was washing. And I couldn't find the words for some things I
was trying to say. My husband had a fit because I wouldn't go to the
hospital. I tried to tell him I was okay, that I knew what it was, and
that I just needed some sleep, but I think I was talking gibberish. He
rang my lovely doctor friends who lived nearby, and they persuaded
me to go to the Coombe. I was grand, but it gave everybody a scare.
Migraine with aura is supposed to get less severe for more than 50 per
cent of pregnant women, but that was not my experience.

People with a history of aura migraine, like I have, may not use the combined contraceptive pill, which contains strong oestrogen, but they can use the progestagen-only pill. The very large, artificially potent molecule of oestrogen in the contraceptive pill, namely ethinylestradiol, is known to be linked to deep vein blood clots. People who have a history of migraine that's preceded by an aura are also a little bit more at risk of getting blood clots, which can lead to ischemic stroke (stroke caused by a clot). The last thing we want to do is put those two risk factors together. So, women with a history of migraine, particularly migraine preceded by an aura, may not use the combined contraceptive pill, patch or ring.

However, because the natural, gentler type of oestrogen that's in transdermal HRT is not linked to blood clots (see Chapter 24), women who have a history of migraine with aura can go on HRT – just like me.

What kind of HRT should you try if you get aura migraine?

There is a lot of confusion among GPs around this topic, and some prescribers worry about starting HRT in women with a history of migraine with aura. However, it is safe to offer HRT to people like us, once everyone understands that we are a special group and that we would like to minimize the impact HRT has on our headache problems.

Some migraine sufferers do better on a steady delivery of oestrogen and progestagen, such as we get in a patch. Others find this sets off their migraine and they fare better on a daily 'shot' of oestrogen, like we get with the spray and the gels.

Dosage also plays a role, with some people tolerating only very small doses of oestrogen before the headache kicks in. The choice of progestagen is important as well: a non-androgenic progestagen – usually our beloved micronized progesterone (P4) – seems to have a better impact on migraine. A Mirena coil can sometimes work, too.

Be prepared for some trial and error. You may need to be prepared to carry your chosen migraine meds around with you and to expect a certain flare up of migraine activity until you finally find the right combo and delivery option for your HRT – and your head. A certain amount of fortitude will be required to eventually find your best cocktail of HRT hormone, and while it's likely to be a case of two steps forward, one step back, you will get there.

Professor Anne MacGregor is a well-known and well-respected UK migraine expert and a member of the British Menopause Society (BMS) advisory group. She also co-authored a book on contraception with my hero, Professor John Guillebaud (see Chapter 5). I recommend that you visit her website at www.annemacgregor.com or get one of her books on migraine and menopause if you want to learn more.

KEY TAKEAWAYS

- ☒ Headache, including migraine headache, may be made worse or better by menopause.
- ☒ HRT may help or HRT may exacerbate headache – it is trial and error sometimes.
- ☒ Migraine preceded by an aura is a risk factor for clots and stroke, therefore sufferers are not allowed to use oestrogen + progestagen contraceptives for this reason.
- ☒ Using HRT is not contraindicated among aura migraine sufferers – you just need to be careful in the formulations you try.

26. Lupus and menopause

Lupus – or, to give it its full name, systemic lupus erythematosus – is a complex auto-immune disease that can range from mild to devastating, and it can affect almost every part of your body. Systemic means 'in the blood', *lupus* means 'wolf' (when first described, many centuries ago, the rash lupus sufferers often get on their face was said to look like they had been bitten by a wolf – I don't know what way wolves like to bite people's faces, but who am I to argue with ancient medical text?) and *erythematosus* means 'redness' or 'inflamed looking'.

The facial rash many people get with lupus looks like two butterfly's wings, one across each cheek, and we call it a malar (meaning jaw) rash. The rash occurs when the body's own immune cells start attacking healthy tissue, which can result in inflammation of varying degrees to organs and systems all over the body. It can be mild and need only minimal lifestyle and pain relief treatments, or it can be severe and lead to chronic disability and early death. It often affects the joints, causing a form of arthritis, but you can also get fevers, the classic butterfly face rash, fatigue and pain.

Diagnosing lupus usually involves suspecting you might have it, first of all, and then doing some blood tests. A positive level of anti-nuclear antibodies (ANA) usually means that your immune system is going on the attack against your own, healthy tissue. We can get a false positive ANA level, though, so the diagnosis needs to be confirmed by a rheumatology specialist.

Lupus can affect your heart, lungs, kidneys, brain (sometimes causing seizures), the blood cells and the gastrointestinal tract. It can flare up and then go into remission. It is incurable, but it is manageable for most people with a range of lifestyle supports and medications – some benign, such as occasional non-steroidal anti-inflammatory meds like ibuprofen and antimalarials (hydroxychloroquine). In other cases, it

needs big-ticket more powerful meds, like corticosteroids and im-
munosuppressive medicines.

Most auto-immune diseases are more likely to be found in women
as opposed to men – we don't know why this is, but it might be something to do with female hormones? This is particularly the case with
lupus as younger women are nine times more likely to be diagnosed
with lupus than men of the same age, so it is suggested that having
female hormones is connected to lupus. It has also been noted that
lupus can improve as women stop having menstrual cycles, which
means the severity of lupus may reduce after menopause.

We must also mention a complication of lupus, known as anti-
phospholipid syndrome (APS). This affects 1 in 5 people with lupus,
and we call it 'secondary' APS then, because it happens alongside
and in conjunction with your lupus. If you have APS all on its own,
without having lupus or any other autoimmune condition, we call it
'primary' APS.

People with APS create antibodies to the phospholipids in their
body. Anti-phospholipid antibodies attack the proteins that bind to
the lipids that help make up your cell walls. They can also affect some
of the many molecules involved in the clotting systems of the blood.
People who have had thrombosis should always be checked for lupus
and APS.

Some people have the AP antibodies but never get a blood clot, so
treatment will depend on whether you are found to be at higher risk
of thrombosis. In general, treatment involves putting you on blood
thinners (aspirin, warfarin, NOACs, DOACs, et cetera) and trying
to avoid things that increase thrombosis risk.

Menopause treatments
for those with lupus

There is a link between premature menopause and lupus in women,
and POI is more common in women with lupus. In fact, some of the
symptoms of the perimenopause are very like some of the symptoms
of mild lupus. And some of the treatments for moderate to severe
lupus create their own problems, particularly osteoporosis and cardiac

disease. All of this must be taken into account when choosing HRT if you have lupus.

Since we know that being a female of reproductive age is a risk factor for lupus, you would imagine that using additional female hormones (especially oestrogen) would make lupus worse. Reassuringly, there have been documented studies where people with lupus used the strong, artificially potent oestrogen present in the contraceptive pill and they seemed to do okay – there was no worsening of their lupus, which suggests that HRT may well be suitable.

While it is not a good idea to use the contraceptive pill if you are someone at higher risk of thrombosis (absolutely no pill if you also have APS), there are lots of non-oestrogen contraceptives you can opt for if you have lupus and/or APS.

When it comes to HRT, while we are always extra cautious when offering it to women with a diagnosis of lupus, there is a very good chance you will be able to try it. Ideally, your HRT choice and management should be shared between a menopause specialist and your lupus specialist, working together. The non-oral varieties of oestrogen are recommended. These should be less risky than the oestrogen contained in the pill as they are more 'body-identical'. The dose should be very low, and you should always use a gel, patch or spray oestrogen, to avoid affecting your risk of blood clots. Your prescriber should also try to get you on natural progesterone (if you need the two hormones), as progesterone is also more 'physiological', i.e. a chemical that the body is already used to.

KEY TAKEAWAYS

- Lupus is a complex auto-immune disease that can affect any part of the body.
- It is more common in menstruating women than post-menopausal women so may be related to ovarian hormone levels.
- HRT is not contraindicated in women with lupus, but HRT choice and management should be shared between a meno-pause specialist and your lupus specialist, working together where possible – particularly if you also have anti-phospholipid syndrome (APS).

27. Managing menopause with HIV

People with human immunodeficiency viruses (HIV) often have additional challenges compared to others when it comes to keeping healthy. People living with HIV are just as likely to experience peri/menopause symptoms as people without HIV. In fact, some research suggests that people living with HIV may be likely to experience menopause symptoms at a younger age and more severely. They may be more exposed to certain chronic medical conditions as a result of their HIV status. Common health problems we usually associate with aging seem to happen earlier (more rapidly) for people living with HIV – this is sometimes called 'accelerated aging'. Also, some of the more common drugs used to treat HIV (known as the 'antiretroviral' class of drugs) may contribute to this accelerated aging. Although modern HIV antiretroviral drugs are more effective and less toxic than 'old school' antiretrovirals, they still may have effects on an aging body that doctors don't fully understand.

It may be that simply having the virus in one's body leads to many of the chronic medical conditions associated with aging. HIV lowers the ability of the immune system to fight off infections; this is often referred to as the immune system being suppressed. In a person living with HIV, the immune system is always struggling to get rid of the virus, so that system is always activated, or 'switched on'. After many years of being constantly activated, the immune system may show signs of premature (too early) aging. In addition, an activated immune system produces inflammation. Ongoing inflammation seems to be related to many conditions, including heart disease and cancer.

People living with HIV also have a higher risk of developing fractures and osteoporosis, kidney and metabolic disorders, neurological problems and heart and liver disease. For these reasons, people with HIV should be prioritized when it comes to mid-life health screening.

The 2018 PRIME (Positive tRansItions through MenopausE) study out of University College London (UCL) recorded data from almost 900 mid-life women with HIV in the UK, most of whom were on antiretroviral medications. This is a very valuable survey as it explores the experience of menopause for HIV+ women and their attitudes towards and use of HRT.

The benefits of HRT for women with HIV

The relationship between oestrogen loss and HIV is grossly under-evaluated. Since we know that menopause is linked to increased risk of certain chronic conditions, such as osteoporosis, and we also know that women with HIV are at greater risk of osteoporosis, there's clearly a benefit to be gained by exploring HRT as a first-line osteoporosis prevention medication for women with HIV who are experiencing menopause symptoms. Similarly, we know that heart disease is more common as we age, especially as our oestrogen levels decline. Women living with HIV are more likely to experience heart attack and stroke, according to the PRIME study. So, the potential benefit of starting oestrogen around the time of your last period to help slow down the development of heart disease (see Chapter 17) goes double for women with HIV.

To me the most striking feature of the PRIME study was how few of the respondents were using any form of hormone replacement. One explanation might be that the women surveyed did not know they were in the peri/menopause. Some of the side effects of their HIV medications were not unlike perimenopause symptoms – fatigue, low mood, anxiety, sleep disruption. Another factor might be sociological or cultural. The majority of the participants in this UCL survey were from Africa, and the study authors suggested that some women from certain African communities were less likely to openly discuss their menopause symptoms than others.

The authors also suggested that the doctors involved did not seem to know who was in charge of sorting out the menopause symptoms. The GP told the ladies to go to the HIV clinic for menopause care, and the HIV services bounced them right back to the GP (sounds familiar!).

HRT can be used while you are taking antiretroviral drugs. Although it would make sense to steer clear of the oral oestrogens that go straight from the stomach to the liver. Stick to patches/gels/sprays to avoid this first whip around that organ. When it comes to the progestagen, the choice is yours. You might go for something like a Mirena coil that gives contraception as well, or you might opt for the gentler, weaker micronized progesterone. There are no conflicts or interactions that have ever been documented between HRT and antiretroviral medications, but antiretroviral drugs in general can and do interfere with lots of other medications, so a good drug interaction check is key.

It has been suggested that some people on HIV medications are reluctant to take even more medications, and that's why they aren't keen on HRT. That is understandable but also, to some extent, sad because we know the many benefits of balancing and supplementing ovarian hormones.

As in all things medical, information is key and the PRIME study authors mentioned an excellent information resource for people with HIV who are starting their menopause journey. See www.aidsmap.com/about-hiv/menopause-and-hiv.

KEY TAKEAWAYS

- If you have HIV, it's very important that you receive comprehensive mid-life screening because you might also be more at risk for aging-related heart, kidney and bone problems *and* your menopause symptoms might start at a younger age than other women.
- Oestrogen can be very beneficial for those with HIV as it helps to lower the risk of heart attack and possibly stroke, both higher risk factors for women with HIV.
- It is safe to use HRT with antiretroviral drugs – but opt for transdermal oestrogen and a progestagen that suits you. Local vaginal oestrogen is also a good idea.

A whole new chapter

Well, that's most of it. That's what I know about the menopause and how to manage it. I hope there was something in here for you and that you have a sense of what you can do for yourself when the time comes or, indeed, if you're already in the middle of it.

Up to relatively recently, menopause hasn't been a common topic of conversation, not anything like the way it is now. But these days you can't look at your phone or read a magazine without seeing a mention of the menopause somewhere – and that is a good thing. All those old stereotypes about 'The Change' are being thrown out, and people are now talking honestly and openly about what it's really like for them and their loved ones.

In the introduction I mentioned Joe Duffy's amazing series of *Liveline* shows about the menopause. As I wrap up here, I want to acknowledge how game-changing that conversation was, as was the subsequent RTÉ One TV documentary *The Change – Ireland's Menopause Story*. These big media moments truly felt like turning points to me. The *Liveline* shows were prompted by a simple email from the wonderful Sallyanne Brady talking about the shortcomings of menopause care in Ireland (Sallyanne is a menopause mentor who co-founded the website theirishmenopause.com). Sallyanne's email tapped into a deep well of suffering and confusion – and also demonstrated that many women were at a complete loss as to how to understand themselves, how to speak to their health-care provider about what they were experiencing, how to get a diagnosis, how to move forward and live their lives. It was so sad and so raw, and it was galvanizing.

The response to that email was a tsunami, so much so that the show had to set up, for the first time, a separate phone line just to deal with the volume of queries. Here is a brilliant description of what went out on the air from *The Irish Times'* Jennifer O'Connell.

Hot flushes, tinnitus, mysterious body pains, joint aches, sore feet, migraines, vertigo, brain fog, forgetfulness, anxiety, digestive issues, insomnia, exhaustion, depression, apathy, isolation, loneliness, cognitive issues, weight gain, lack of sex drive, even suicidal ideation. One woman likened herself to a slow puncture. One felt as though she hit a brick wall. Another said it was like being hit by an exploding bomb. Caller after caller said they knew something was wrong, they just never associated it with menopause. Many had never heard of perimenopause, the years leading up to menopause in which many punishing symptoms come crashing into women's lives.

I was oblivious to the radio discussion when it first started. I was out on my regular weekly hill walk and got a text: 'They are talking about menopause on *Liveline* and some of the callers are mentioning your name.'

I immediately thought, *I have said something stupid and am in trouble* – I often do and I often am – so I listened back on the RTÉ Player that night and to my amazement I discovered Joe Duffy and team had done that day's full show on the menopause, and it was the second in a row (the show ending up devoting an unprecedented eight days to the topic). I was so pleased that the menopause was getting so much airtime (and that I was not in trouble!), but I did hear some information that I thought wasn't completely accurate. So, being a bit of a know-it-all, I decided to text the show and set them right. The next day, the producers had me at the end of the line, dealing with some questions.

The conversation continued into the following week and one of the producers contacted me asking if I could come into the studio. I did not know it then, but realized after, that it is a rare privilege to be invited into the studio to join Joe in person – it is a call-in show, after all. We took calls from many women and their loved ones, and heard so many stories – some funny, some heartbreaking – and it was a good day. I must have been more affected by the experience than I realized because I turned left for home, instead of right to go towards the city centre, and forgot all about being on duty in Holles Street that afternoon.

The TV documentary in 2022 was sensitive, powerful and optimistic – exactly what you want when dealing with menopause.

It allowed women to tell their own stories, which gave everyone a clearer and more detailed picture of what this time of life feels like for the person going through it. I think that's really important. When the media follows this line, it leads to greater empathy and insight, which helps everyone, from the women themselves to us doctors and prescribers. And I think people did listen.

All of this is for the good. It takes away the sense of mystery and fear that used to shroud mid-life's physical changes, and it makes everyone feel like it's just a normal part of life – which is exactly what it is. Much as I welcome the media's embrace of a healthy attitude towards discussing the menopause, I'm conscious that the mood can change, just as it did in 2002 around the publication of the WHI study. So, do not act on health information from the media. Get a GP you trust, someone who embraces your concerns openly, and they will be your safe place for advice.

Does everyone have a horrible menopause transition?
No.
Does everyone need to go on HRT?
No.
Most people do grand all on their own. They might take stock and do things to improve their diet, activity, smoking and drinking habits. They might start going for routine screening check-ups and take advice from a trusted GP. Whatever is best for you.

If you're in perimenopause, first do whatever you can to help yourself with regard to living healthier and being kinder to yourself. Then be reassured that there is plenty of help for you if you are experiencing tough symptoms. Things are really getting better for women, and there is more discussion and research going on right now. Do not accept misery. Get whatever help is out there. You do not have to do this alone.

If you're too young to be hitting any of this yet, please do not fear for your future. Try to make good lifestyle choices NOW, get your exercise, eat your greens, go easy on the booze and do not smoke – lay down some good groundwork for your body's lifetime health.

Some people will really struggle with menopause, and for those who do, there are medical treatments and therapies out there. Have a look online at any of the many excellent and free Irish and UK websites that discuss prescription and non-prescription therapies for HRT (there's a list of resources on pages 295–6). If you do not have any major contraindications to HRT use and you want to try it, try it. But be patient, HRT is not a panacea – it's just a little help where it's needed.

This is easy to say, of course, if you are not battling cancer or a chronic disease, where the treatments involved can put you at risk of future disease. Not everyone is a candidate for hormone supplements, and some do not want them. You are not 'less than' if you do not need HRT, choose not to take HRT or have been told to avoid HRT.

If there is no family history of anything that prevents you trying HRT, it is a safe option – much, much safer than the contraceptive pill. Tell your GP you want to try it and if they are not willing to let you do so, ask them what guidelines they are using to deny you access to it.

Let's face it, aging isn't fun, but the alternative is worse, and now we older women can look forward to our second act without necessarily being plunged into awful symptoms and decrepitude. But there's more to aging well than just slapping on a HRT patch! The second fifty years of our lives can be positive and empowering – just think: period-free, pregnancy-free, kids getting set up elsewhere – this is OUR time. Stop thinking, 'What needs to be done?' and start thinking, 'What do I want to do?' And do it. I hope this book will not just inform you but help you to feel empowered and optimistic about the years ahead.

When US gynaecologist Dr Robert Wilson published his 1966 book *Feminine Forever* (promoting the benefits of menopausal oestrogen therapy), he got some negative press, particularly from many feminist groups. I understand their dismay; I don't feel the need to be 'feminine' forever, thank you very much, Robert! But I would like to avoid preventable diseases and enjoy a good quality of life. I want to be able to work until I choose to stop, to chase a grandchild without getting chest pain or breaking my hip, and to enjoy every day I am granted. Now, that's not too much to ask, wouldn't you say?

Acknowledgements

When I was approached to do this book, my initial reaction was, *No way. That will be way too much work* – and it was! But now I am glad we did it, and I have to thank my task mistress, editor Rachel Pierce, for being so patient with me. I also want to thank Patricia Deevy for asking me to write the book and being there every step of the way. The whole Penguin team have provided fantastic support – it was a challenge, but we got there!

This book is about the menopause; what effect it could have on you and what you need to know when deciding how to cope with it. The biggest secret of managing your menopause is not in this book, though. It is the same secret ingredient that applies to all the hurdles that life throws at us – family and friends.

I don't know how things would have been without the blessing of good friends and my amazing family. My weekly hikes with Áine and Aisling have helped me gain some fitness and some sanity! *Go raibh maith agaibh* for the cheap psychotherapy, ladies!

I am disorganized and lazy. I get some good ideas and then get distracted by hoovering or playing 15 x 15 square Sudokus that take two hours. I rely heavily on the support of my colleagues/friends and would never have been able to make my contribution to menopause education and care without lots of help. Dr Nicola Cochrane, in particular, has been an enormous part of the menopause journey in Ireland and could easily have been the subject of her own TV show if she was more of a ham – like me. She does what so many GPs do in Ireland, which is to keep up to date and manage all the work of general practice while simultaneously offering the best possible information and advice to menopausal patients. Thank you, Nicola, for all you've done and all you're gonna do because we are only getting started! With her support and the hard work of our team in the menopause clinic in Holles Street, I think the best is yet to come.

Dr Brian Kennedy (whom I often refer to as 'Worshipful Master of the Menopause') is another GP who makes offering menopause care in general practice look easy (it isn't). He is the mastermind behind the Telegram instant message group known as 'HRT Prescribers'. This is a doctor-only app for medics who strive to do their best for menopausal patients. Brian has over 800 people on there, sharing information on menopause and HRT every single day. *Maith thú*, Brian!

I also need to send a shout-out to my long-time friend/GP colleague/educational-meeting-travel-companion-and-roommate/neighbour/walking pal and all-round good person, Dr Geraldine Holland. It was her invitation that got me started as a teacher in women's health and started me on this journey that I hope will last as long as my brain does. Our most common texts just say 'Walk?' Long may that last!

My family is spread across two continents.

Most of my Lundys are still on Long Island (in New York), where I grew up. I see them all the time – I go there, they come here – but when I arrived in Ireland in 1978, I had no one. People were so kind – Ireland was and is a very friendly country and I made loads of friends – but I did not have any family of my own. Until I met my husband's family. For the last forty years, the Magees have been my Irish family. Hogan's mam, Eileen, and his dad, Ted, looked after me like I was one of their own and I can't imagine where I would have landed without their kindness. I am eternally grateful to them for that. My sister-in-law, Mairéad, and her husband, Philip, and their wonderful children, Tighernán, Sunni and Seoinín, are some of the sweetest, kindest, most loving humans you will ever meet. It is a privilege to be the kids' auntie! Mairéad (Raidy to us) claims she learned lots of her parenting skills from me. Jeez, I hope not – *she* is a mom you'd be lucky to have.

In New York, my mom, Mary, still rules the roost at eighty-seven years of age – stirring up the s★★t and causing all kinds of trouble. She is an inspiration on how to age not so much gracefully as on your own terms! She misses my dad – we all do – he died in 2013, at ninety-one years of age. John Joseph Lundy Sr. was one of a kind – not always the easiest person to live with, to be fair, but full of love, and an inspirational teacher and talker – we have all inherited that from him. May you have as interesting a life as my mom and dad.

My sisters, Noreen and Rosanna, and my brother, John (who lives in a castle in Cork now!) are close. My sisters stayed together when I went away, they see each other every week and their kids are more like siblings than cousins. They (we) fight like a bag of cats sometimes – what Irish family doesn't? – but we are always there for one another, without question, without hesitation. They allow me to swan about and take over their lives every time I swoop in for a visit. I take that for granted 'cause I think I am delightful! To them I apologize, and pray we have many more years of bugging each other.

My own immediate family are, of course, my life.

My husband, Hogan, and my children, Murchadh, Seán and Nóra, were my vocation. I always wanted to be a doctor but never full-time, because I wanted to be a wife and mom first and foremost. I have been rewarded with some of the best human beings anyone could meet. Hogan has been with me for over forty years and while a family business limited his day-to-day activities with me and the kids when they were younger, he made up for it by being a dad of infinite kindness, patience and understanding. The kids and I have been truly blessed. I am lucky to have him as my husband and the father of my children.

Mur and Seán are good boys and wonderful sons and they love their Mammy – the way I taught them to! They were always open to a bribe and I could get them to accompany me on hikes once the promise of good food and maybe a PlayStation game was in the offing. Without any actual input on my part, they have embraced what it means to be a modern man. That is, someone who embodies masculinity through both strength and gentleness, without being threatened by strong female energies (me!). I am proud of the people they have become, but the credit is all their own, with a sprinkling of their dad for good measure.

Lastly, I need to mention my queen, my angel, my daughter, Nóra. She has had to endure me and my moods and my drama for longer than most people – and she has survived. She deserves a medal for that alone. She has been dragged along on countless hikes and walks with our evil dachshund, Denny, and his sidekick, the now sixteen-year-old 'Pet Cemetery' alumnus, Buddy – the ugliest, dumbest, sweetest dog – and Nóra has only complained a little. We have also worked together for many years. She agreed to join in as one of my team of 'simulated patients' when I used to do live training for GPs in sexual health. The poor kid is immortalized on videos all over Ireland as 'Teenager with the weird STI' or 'Young woman who has side effects from the pill'. Looking back now, this might have been a form of child abuse – sorry, Nóra! She has taught me loads about love and communication and just being a woman in the twenty-first century. The person she has become radiates love and acceptance and intelligence, and this is not because of me, but in spite of me. I am in awe. *Grá mo chroí*.

Sources of further information

Online sources

www.annemacgregor.com: a specialist in headache and women's health

www.arccancersupport.ie: comprehensive support services for people with cancer and their families

www.bma.org.uk: the British Medical Association (BMA)

www.daisynetwork.org: website of the UK-based Daisy Network, a well-known and highly respected POI support organization

www.emas-online.org: the European Menopause and Andropause Society (EMAS)

www.imsociety.org: the International Menopause Society (IMS)

www.managemymenopause.co.uk: tailored lifestyle advice for the menopause

www.menopause.org.au: the Australasian Menopause Society (AMS)

www.menopausematters.co.uk: independent website providing up-to-date information

www.menopausesupport.co.uk: for video blogs about all aspects of the menopause

www.nice.org.uk: the UK's National Institute for Health and Care Excellence (NICE)

www.nmh.ie: for information on the Complex Menopause Clinic at the National Maternity Hospital, Holles Street

www.thebms.org.uk: the British Menopause Society (BMS)
- go to **thebms.org.uk/publications/bms-tv/** to view short videos explaining aspects of the menopause

www.theirishmenopause.com and **theirish_menopause** Instagram page: both hosted by menopause mentor Sallyanne Brady

www.themenopausecharity.org: for help from menopause specialist Dr Louise Newson

www.womens-health-concern.org: for factsheets and advice from the patient arm of the BMS

Books

There are thousands of books, but I recommend these.

Abernathy, Kathy. 2018. *Menopause: The One-Stop Guide*. London: Profile

Hilliard, Tim et al. 2021. *Management of the Menopause* (6th edition) aka *The BMS Handbook*. Marlow: BMS Publications Ltd

Newson, Dr Louise. 2021. *Preparing for the Perimenopause and Menopause*. London: Penguin Books

Panay, Nicholas et al. (eds). 2020. *Managing the Menopause* (2nd edition). Cambridge: Cambridge University Press

Short, Dr Hannah, and Leonhardt, Dr Mandy. 2002. *The Complete Guide to POI and Early Menopause*. London: Sheldon Press

For medical practitioners –
key sources used in this book

Online sources

Australian Menopause Society. Information sheet 'Bleeding – perimenopausal, postmenopausal and breakthrough bleeding on MHT/ HRT'. Last updated March 2017: https://www.menopause.org.au/ images/stories/infosheets/docs/AMS_Peri_and_postmenopausal_bleed ing_including_breakthrough_on_MHT.pdf

British Menopause Society. Consensus statement on non-hormonal-based treatments for menopausal symptoms. Reviewed June 2022: https://thebms.org.uk/publications/consensus-statements/non-hormonal-based-treatments-menopausal-symptoms/

British Menopause Society. Tool for clinicians 'Progestogens and endometrial protection'. Published October 2021: https://thebms.org.uk/wp-content/ uploads/2021/10/14-BMS-TfC-Progestogens-and-endometrial-protection-01H.pdf

British Menopause Society. Consensus statement on premature ovarian insufficiency. Reviewed April 2020: https://thebms.org.uk/publications/ consensus-statements/premature-ovarian-insufficiency/

European Society of Human Reproduction & Embryology (ESHRE). 'Guideline on the management of premature ovarian insufficiency'. Published December 2015: https://www.eshre.eu/Guidelines-and-Legal/ Guidelines/Management-of-premature-ovarian-insufficiency.aspx

International Menopause Society (IMS). Position papers and consensus statements, 2019-21: https://www.imsociety.org/statements/position-papers-and-consensus-statements/

National Institute for Health and Care Excellence (NICE). Guideline NG23. 'Menopause: diagnosis and management'. Published 12 November 2015, last updated 5 December 2019: https://www.nice.org.uk/guidance/ng23

Primary Care Women's Health Forum. 'How to manage women presenting with abnormal uterine bleeding in primary care without face to
face contact'. Reviewed March 2021: https://pcwhf.co.uk/wp-content/
uploads/2020/04/PWCHF-HMB-without-face-to-face-contact.pdf

Articles, reports, papers

Cold, S. et al. 2022. 'Systemic or vaginal hormone therapy after early breast
cancer: A Danish observational cohort study'. *Journal of the National Cancer
Institute*. Online publication 20 July: https://doi.org/10.1093/jnci/djac112

Collaborative Group on Hormonal Factors in Breast Cancer. 2019. 'Type and
timing of menopausal hormone therapy and breast cancer risk: individual participant meta-analysis of the worldwide epidemiological evidence'.
Lancet, 394 (10204), 1159–68

Collins, P. et al. 2016. 'Cardiovascular risk assessment in women – an update'.
Climacteric, 19 (4), 329–36

Dubey, R. K. et al. 2004. 'Hormone replacement therapy and cardiovascular
disease: what went wrong and where do we go from here?' *Hypertension*,
44 (6), 789–95

Fournier, A. et al. 2008. 'Unequal risks for breast cancer associated with
different hormone replacement therapies: results from the E3N cohort
study'. *Breast Cancer Research and Treatment*, 107 (1), 103–11

Furness, S. et al. 2009. 'Hormone therapy in postmenopausal women and
risk of endometrial hyperplasia'. *Cochrane Database of Systematic Reviews*,
15 (2): CD000402

Hamoda, H. et al. 2016. 'The British Menopause Society & Women's Health
Concern 2016 recommendations on hormone replacement therapy in
menopausal women'. *Post Reproductive Health*, 22 (4), 165–83

Jane, F. M. & Davis, S. R. 2014. 'A practitioner's toolkit for managing the
menopause'. *Climacteric*, 17 (5) 564–79

Kendall, A. et al. 2006. 'Caution: vaginal estradiol appears to be contraindicated in postmenopausal women on adjuvant aromatase inhibitors'. *Annals
of Oncology*, 17 (4), 584–7

Khalil, R. A. 2013. 'Estrogen, vascular estrogen receptor and hormone therapy in postmenopausal vascular disease'. *Biochemical Pharmacology*, 86 (12),
1627–42

Kim, C. et al. 2015. 'A review of the relationships between endogenous sex steroids and incident ischemic stroke and coronary heart disease events'. *Current Cardiology Reviews*, 11 (3), 252–60

Lambrinoudaki, I. et al. 2021. 'Premature ovarian insufficiency: a toolkit for the primary care physician'. *Climacteric*, 24 (5), 425–37

Mariani, L. et al. 2013. 'Vaginal atrophy in breast cancer survivors: role of vaginal estrogen therapy'. *Gynecological Endocrinology*, 29 (1), 25–9

Million Women Study Collaborators. 2002.'Patterns of use of hormone replacement therapy in one million women in Britain, 1996–2000'. *BJOG International Journal of Obstetrics and Gynaecology*, 109 (12), 1319–30

Mosca, L. et al. 2011. 'Sex/gender differences in cardiovascular disease prevention: what a difference a decade makes'. *Circulation*, 124 (19), 2145–54.

Panay, N. et al. 2013. 'The 2013 British Menopause Society & Women's Health Concern recommendations on hormone replacement therapy'. *Menopause International*, 19 (2), 59–68

Renoux, C. et al. 2010. 'Hormone replacement therapy and the risk of venous thromboembolism: a population-based study'. *Journal of Thrombosis and Haemostasis*, 8 (5), 979–86

Rosenthal, T & Oparil, S. 2000. 'Hypertension in women'. *Journal of Human Hypertension*, 14 (10-11), 691–704

Streff, A. et al. 2021. 'Changes in serum estradiol levels with Estring in postmenopausal women with breast cancer treated with aromatase inhibitors'. *Support Care Cancer*, 29 (1), 187–91

Upton, C. E. et al. 2021. 'Premature ovarian insufficiency: the need for evidence on the effectiveness of hormonal therapy'. *Climacteric*, 24 (5), 453–8

Vinogradova, Y. 2020. 'Use of hormone replacement therapy and risk of breast cancer: nested case-control studies using the QResearch and CPRD databases'. *British Medical Journal*, 371: m3873

Notes

1. What is the menopause?

p. 6 **'menopause, like big brains and upright posture'**: Dr Jared Diamond quoted in Natalie Angier, 'Theorists See Evolutionary Advantages in Menopause', *New York Times*, 16 September 1997.

p. 7 **becoming post-menopausal is a relatively new phenomenon**: if you'd like to read more on this, see Pollycove, R. et al. 2011. 'The evolutionary origin and significance of menopause'. *Menopause*, 18 (3), 336–42.

2. How will you know?

p. 20 **there has been some useful research conducted into the timeline**: SWAN is an ongoing US project, started in 1996, that was designed to define the menopause transition and to lay out its characteristics and consequences – both biologically and psychosocially – for an ethnically and racially diverse population (Black, Chinese, Hispanic, Japanese and white). The study examined menopause symptoms and mental health, sleep, bone, body composition, cardiovascular risks, physical functions, cognitive performance and vaginal and urogenital health.

p. 20 **2001 Stages of Reproductive Aging Workshop**: STRAW is another USA-based initiative trying to identify a staging system for perimenopause, menopause and ovarian aging. The main participants in the STRAW group include the National Institute on Aging (NIA) (part of the National Institutes of Health (NIH)), the Office of Research on Women's Health (ORWH), the North American Menopause Society (NAMS), the American Society for Reproductive Medicine (ASRM), the International Menopause Society (IMS) and the US Endocrine Society. The STRAW group met again in

2011, ten years after commencing, to revise their perimenopause-to-menopause-to-post-menopause timeline. They sensibly called that paper STRAW +10. See Harlow, S. D. et al. 2012. 'Executive summary of the Stages of Reproductive Aging Workshop +10: addressing the unfinished agenda of staging reproductive aging'. *Menopause*, 19 (4), 387–95.

5. The good news – you don't have to put up with vaginal symptoms

p. 48 **the symptoms of GSM can all be helped**: information in this chapter (and previously Chapter 4) is sourced from the 2017 *Guidance on diagnosis and management of urogenital atrophy or genitourinary syndrome of the menopause (GSM)* from the Primary Care Women's Health Forum and the BMS handbook *Management of the Menopause* (6th edition, revised 2021). See also the NICE guidelines 'Menopause: diagnosis and management' (2015, updated 2019).

p. 52 **There is a small, often quoted study**: Kendall, A. et al. 2006. 'Caution: vaginal estradiol appears to be contraindicated in postmenopausal women on adjuvant aromatase inhibitors'. *Annals of Oncology*, 17 (4), 584–7.

6. Early onset menopause arising from hormone issues

p. 58 **A recent study of more than 11,000 Australians**: Xu, X. et al. 2020. 'Age at natural menopause and development of chronic conditions and multimorbidity: results from an Australian prospective cohort'. *Human Reproduction*, 35 (1), 203–11; also Podfigurna-Stopa, A. et al. 2016. 'Premature ovarian insufficiency: the context of long-term effects'. *Journal of Endocrinological Investigation*, 39 (9), 983–90.

p. 58 **Genetic disorders that can be linked to POI**: many POI ladies tell me they struggle to find good medical information. Sheldon Press in the UK have recently published a new book by Dr Hannah Short and Dr Mandy Leonhardt (in June 2022), *The Complete Guide to POI and Early Menopause*. It gives detailed information on POI, Turner Syndrome and Fragile X.

p. 61 **it is highly recommended to use some form of replacement sex hormones**: according to the BMS consensus statement on the management of women with premature ovarian insufficiency: https://thebms.org.uk/publications/consensus-statements/premature-ovarian-insufficiency/. See also the European Society of Human Reproduction and Embryology (ESHRE) 2015 guidelines on POI: www.eshre.eu/Guidelines-and-Legal/Guidelines/Management-of-premature-ovarian-insufficiency.aspx.

8. Non-HRT treatment options for menopause symptoms

p. 90 **BMS guidelines on non-hormonal treatments**: https://thebms.org.uk/publications/consensus-statements/non-hormonal-based-treatments-menopausal-symptoms/.

10. Oestrogen – the caped superhero!

p. 107 **could even reverse this process**: Sassarini, J. & Lumsden, M. A. 2015. 'Oestrogen replacement in postmenopausal women'. *Age and Ageing*, 44 (4), 551–8.

p. 108 **There are a number of suspected benefits**: Fait, T. 2019. 'Menopause hormone therapy: latest developments and clinical practice'. *Drugs in Context*, 8: 212551.

p. 113 **none of this is definitive as of yet**: Fournier et al. 2008. 'Unequal risks for breast cancer associated with different hormone replacement therapies: results from the E3N cohort study'. *Breast Cancer Research and Treatment*, 107 (1), 103–11.

p. 115 **women who already have increased risk of clotting problems**: Vinogradova, Y. et al. 2019. 'Use of hormone replacement therapy and risk of venous thromboembolism: nested case-control studies using the QResearch and CPRD databases'. *British Medical Journal*, 364: k4810.

p. 115 **try micronized progesterone or the dydrogesterone progestagens, in combination with transdermal estradiol**: Viscoli, C. M. et al. 2001. 'A clinical trial of oestrogen-replacement therapy after ischemic stroke'. *New England Journal of Medicine*, 345 (17), 1243–9.

11. Progestagen — the yin to oestrogen's yang

p. 120 **more work is needed before P4 replaces the oestrogen in HRT, but it is a potentially exciting development**: Prior, J. C. 2018. 'Progesterone for treatment of symptomatic menopausal women'. *Climacteric*, 21 (4), 358–65.

12. Testosterone — the trusty sidekick

p. 128 **A blood test must be done to measure the amount of testosterone in the blood**: for clinicians reading this, section 7 of the BMS *Tools for Clinicians. Testosterone assays — interpretation of results* advises: 'Although it is not mandatory to perform testosterone level estimation prior to or for monitoring treatment, it can be useful. A low FAI < 1.0% in women with symptoms of low sexual desire and arousal supports the use of testosterone supplementation. Repeat estimation at the 2–3 month follow up visit can be performed to demonstrate if there has been an increase in levels, though clinical response is of paramount importance. It is also useful to demonstrate that values are being maintained within the female physiological range, typically < 5.0%, thus making androgenic side effects less likely.'

p. 129 **It is licensed for the treatment of low libido in menopause**: Davis, S. R. et al. 2019. 'Global consensus position statement on the benefits of testosterone therapy for women'. *Climacteric*, 22 (5), 429–34.

p. 129 **Some studies have shown benefits on the skeleton**: Hamoda, H. et al. 2016. 'The British Menopause Society & Women's Health Concern 2016 recommendations on hormone replacement therapy in menopausal women'. *Post Reproductive Health*, 22 (4), 165–83.

14. Bio-identical (aka body-identical) HRT explained

p. 139 **it's sort of a mix of natural base and synthetic process**: if you are interested to find out more about how hormones are made, I can recommend this excellent article: Julia Kollewe, 'HRT: inside the complex global supply chain behind a \$20bn market', *Guardian*, 24 September 2022.

p. 139 **it's a crazy, complicated chemical process**: Jackson, L. M. et al. (eds). 2020. *The Clinical Utility of Compounded Bioidentical Hormone Therapy: A Review of Safety, Effectiveness, and Use*. Washington, DC: National Academies Press. See Section 4: 'Reproductive Steroid Hormones: Synthesis, Structure, and Biochemistry'. Available from https://www.ncbi.nlm.nih.gov/books/NBK562873/.

15. HRT and unscheduled bleeding

p. 157 **we need to change your HRT and maybe start to investigate**: for prescribers, here are some options I present to patients: increase the dose or change the type of progestagen; change the progestagen schedule; reduce the dose of oestrogen; try using the progestagen sequentially for three months. For the reasons given in this chapter, stopping HRT should be the last resort, but if the bleed doesn't settle off HRT, it needs investigating. While I feel confident in providing patients with these options because I do it all the time, some of you might feel anxious about playing around with the cocktails – and I don't blame you. We offer suggestions and support for Irish (and, it seems, UK) HRT prescribers on the fabulous 800+ strong Telegram app under 'HRT prescribing GP group' – although what we really need is free, hospital-based advice for HRT users and prescribers, and I am planning to roll that out as part of the Complex Menopause Service at the National Maternity Hospital.

p. 163 **the data do not bear that out**: Moorman, P. G. et al. 2011. 'Effect of hysterectomy with ovarian preservation on ovarian function'. *Obstetrics and Gynecology*, 118 (6), 1271–9.

17. Your heart and the menopause

p. 193 **telling a lady to see her GP about anxiety medication**: Blomkalns, A. L. et al. 2005. 'Gender disparities in the diagnosis and treatment of non-ST-segment elevation acute coronary syndromes: large-scale observations from the CRUSADE (Can Rapid Risk Stratification of Unstable Angina Patients Suppress Adverse Outcomes with Early Implementation of the American College of Cardiology/American Heart Association Guidelines) National Quality Improvement Initiative'. *Journal of the American College of Cardiology*, 45 (6), 832–7.

p. 194 **the many cardiovascular benefits given to us by oestrogen**: Dubey, R. K. et al. 2004. 'Hormone replacement therapy and cardiovascular disease: what went wrong and where do we go from here?' *Hypertension*, 44 (6), 789–95.

p. 194 **carotid intima-media thickness (CIMT)**: Thurston, R. C. et al. 2016. 'Menopausal hot flashes and carotid intima media thickness among midlife women'. *Stroke*, 47 (12), 2910–15; Meer, A. & Kinsara, A. 2021. 'Gender differences in patients presenting with NSTEMI in the STAR registry'. *European Journal of Preventive Cardiology*, 28, Suppl 1.

p. 196 **a French study from about ten years ago**: Scarabin-Carré, V. et al. 2012. 'High level of plasma estradiol as a new predictor of ischemic arterial disease in older postmenopausal women: the three-city cohort study'. *Journal of the American Heart Association*, 1 (3): e001388.

p. 197 **a 2012 Danish study**: Schierbeck, L. L. et al. 2012. 'Effect of hormone replacement therapy on cardiovascular events in recently postmenopausal women: randomized trial'. *British Medical Journal*, 345: e6409.

p. 198 **the Timing Hypothesis of HRT**: this theory is supported by other frequently quoted studies: the Kronos Early Oestrogen Prevention Study (KEEPS) and Early versus Late Intervention Trial with Estradiol (ELITE). See Mehta, J. M. et al. 2019. 'The Timing Hypothesis: hormone therapy for treating symptomatic women during menopause and its relationship to cardiovascular disease'. *Journal of Women's Health (2002)*, 28 (5), 705–11.

p. 198 **a more recent Finnish study**: also Mikkola, T. S., et al. 2015. 'Increased cardiovascular mortality risk in women discontinuing post-menopausal hormone therapy'. *Journal of Clinical Endocrinology and Metabolism*, 100 (12), 4588–94.

p. 199 **we are likely to get symptoms from the vessel disease**: Dubey et al. 'Hormone replacement therapy and cardiovascular disease'.

18. Breast cancer and the menopause

p. 217 **a small, badly controlled UK study**: Kendall, A. et al. 2006. 'Caution: vaginal estradiol appears to be contraindicated in postmenopausal women on adjuvant aromatase inhibitors'. *Annals of Oncology*, 17 (4), 584–7.

p. 217 **a very recently published observational study from Denmark**: Cold, S. et al. 2022. 'Systemic or vaginal hormone therapy after early breast cancer: A Danish observational cohort study'. *Journal of the National Cancer Institute*. Online publication 20 July: https://doi.org/10.1093/jnci/djac112.

p. 218 **there are many others that might also increase your risk**: these include Lynch syndrome (PMS2, MLH1 and MSH2 genes), Cowden syndrome (PTEN gene), Li-Fraumeni syndrome (TP53 gene), Peutz-Jeghers syndrome (STK11 gene), ataxia telangiectasia (ATM gene), hereditary diffuse gastric cancer (CDH1 gene), PALB2 gene and CHEK2 gene.

p. 219 **much higher lifetime risk of breast and ovarian cancer**: Rippy, L. & Marsden, J. 2006. 'Is HRT justified for symptom management in women at higher risk of developing breast cancer?' *Climacteric*, 9 (6), 404–15; also Sellars, T. et al. 1997. 'The role of hormone replacement therapy in the risk for breast cancer and total mortality in women with a family history of breast cancer'. *Annals of Internal Medicine*, 127 (11), 973–80.

p. 220 **use of HRT appears not to *increase* risk:** Rebeck, T. et al. 2005. 'Effect of short-term hormone replacement therapy on breast cancer risk reduction after bilateral prophylactic oophorectomy in BRCA1 and BRCA2 mutation carriers: the PROSE Study Group'. *Journal of Clinical Oncology*, 23 (31), 7804–10; also Eisen, A. et al. 2008. 'Hormone therapy and the risk of breast cancer in BRCA1 mutation carriers'. *Journal of the National Cancer Institute*, 100 (19), 1361–7.

19. Your bones and the menopause

p. 223 **the burden of disability from osteoporosis on the health services**: Johnell, O. & Kanis, J. A. 2006. 'An estimate of the worldwide prevalence and disability associated with osteoporotic fractures'. *Osteoporosis International*, 17 (12), 1726–33.

21. Menopause care for transgender people

p. 249 **give you any information that's available and that might apply specifically to you**: the information in this chapter is based on the guidelines published by the Irish College of General Practitioners. See Crowley, D. & Lacey, V. 2021. *Guide for Providing Care for Transgender Patients in Primary Care*. Quick Reference Guide (Version 2). Dublin: ICGP.

24. Menopause, HRT use and the risk of blood clotting

p. 273 **your risk of blood clots is whatever your own background personal risk is**: Vinogradova, Y. et al. 2019. 'Use of hormone replacement therapy and risk of venous thromboembolism: nested case-control studies using the QResearch and CPRD databases'. *British Medical Journal*, 364: k4810.
p. 274 **a large review of thrombosis and HRT**: ibid.

27. Managing menopause with HIV

p. 284 **The 2018 PRIME (Positive tRansItions through MenopausE) study**: 'Menopause in women living with HIV in England: findings from the PRIME Study' – you can read the full report here: https://www.ucl.ac.uk/global-health/sites/global-health/files/prime-report-2018.pdf.

Epilogue: A whole new chapter

p. 287 **here is a brilliant description of what went out on the air**: Jennifer O'Connell, 'Why don't we want to talk about menopause?', *The Irish Times*, 15 May 2021.